Breast Cancer Chronicles

By Erica J. Holloman, PhD

3

Breast Cancer Chronicles

By Erica J. Holloman, PhD

© 2014 - Josie & Erica Holloman

All rights reserved. No part of this book may be reproduced or transmitted in any form or by any electronic or mechanical means including information storage and retrieval systems, without permission in writing from the authors. The only exception is by a reviewer, who may quote short excerpts in a review to be printed in a magazine, newspaper, or on the Web.

Although the authors and publishers of this book have made every effort to ensure the completeness and accuracy of the information contained in this book, we assume no responsibility for errors, inaccuracies, or omissions contained herein. Any slights of people, places, or organizations are unintentional.

All pictures and cover art provided by The Holloman family and Wagner Wolf, LLC

WagnerWolf.com

ericajhollomanfoundationinc.org

Acknowledgments

First we - Erica and I - want to thank everyone who read Erica's blogs. Blogging allowed Erica to share her inner thoughts and educate along the way.

Gina and Marvin – thank you for always being on call whenever we needed you.

To my best friend LaTasha (who is Erica's godmother) – when Erica passed and I called home, you stepped in and handled things. For that, I am truly grateful.

Calvin - thank you for having our back, no matter what. You are a true friend.

I want to thank my Gestational Carrier (surrogate). A million "Thank You's" will never be enough. I will never forget what you have done for us.

Thanks McKenzie for dropping everything and coming when we called.

Adrian - you know why!

Candis for all the typing and editing.

Juanita for listening to me cry.

I want to thank my husband and Erica's father, Bobby, for loving both of us unconditionally. For driving us up and down the road for chemo appointments, surgeries, and vacations, etc. Lol.

I am thankful for Erica's friends. People say that when someone dies, the communication stops and after a couple of weeks you are all alone. In my case it was exactly 2 ½ years. I talked to one of Erica's friends every day for 985 days straight. I thank each of you for that. These remarkable people started out as supporters and became cherished friends.

Thanks Terez - on my first Mother's Day without Erica you took the time to send me a card before you left the country so I would have it on Mother's Day. It's little things like that that make you special.

Janice, Ebony, Quay, Mona, Leesha, Kisha, Jonathan (JJ), Andrew, Ra'Shawn, and Zaria all started out as friends and now are more like sons and daughters. They are always 'Smiling For Erica'.

I want to thank my niece, Kelly. We became friends; I guess in some way we needed each other.

Thanks Christine for the hookup! Thanks to my publishing company, Wagner Wolf LLC, for believing in Erica's project.

I thank my family, immediate and extended, for all their love and support.

Finally, I want to thank the following Universities and Organizations for their support. The University of Louisville - special thanks to President James R. Ramsey. The faculty and staff of the College of Education and Graduate School. Hey Dr. Cuyjet! Wake Forest University's School of Business faculty, staff, and students for all the love they have shown.

Thanks to Barbee and Shayla for being the first people to convince me to finish the book. Thanks to Dean Steve Reinemund for cutting your vacation short to do Erica's eulogy.

Thanks to the women of Zeta Phi Beta Sorority, Inc. – Pi Sigma Zeta chapter in Forest Park, Ohio. To the men of Phi Beta Sigma Fraternity, Inc. - Lambda Theta Chapter, University of Cincinnati and Delta Theta Sigma Chapter, Cincinnati Alumni. Pan African Network (PAN), a subcommittee of American College

Personnel Association (ACPA), for the continued support of the Erica J Holloman Foundation.

A special Thanks to Candice, MaKayla, Madyson and Morgan for loving us.

Thanks to my mother for loving both me and Erica unconditionally. I want to thank my father (who just recently joined Erica in heaven) for always believing in both of us.

ERICA, I Thank GOD every day for letting me LOVE you for 35 years.

Josie and Erica Holloman

From The Publisher...

Wagner Wolf Publishing welcomes you to "Breast Cancer Chronicles by Erica J. Holloman, PhD". This is the story of a brave young woman, Erica Holloman, and her encounters with the trying disease. This is also a mother's story, where Josephine Holloman, Erica's devoted mother, tells you how it has been to watch a child struggle to survive.

We are humbled and honored to help bring this story to life. We hope we have done justice to Erica's beautiful and heartbreaking journey. We hope we have highlighted the devotion of a mother as she watches her only child deal with deep issues of health, career, family, and love.

This book is based on a blog Erica produced while going through her cancer trials. Each entry will center around a date in Erica's blog, and will have a calendar, drug, and procedure reference to help you follow along. If there is an unfamiliar word or term used, feel free to look it up in our glossary at the end of the book.

Most importantly, enjoy this book! Enjoy the care and honesty contained in these pages. Put yourself in this family's place and explore how you would react to each situation. Hold your loved ones a little tighter. Be grateful for the blessings and miracles in your life. Join the fight against breast cancer to save lives and ease the sting of this cruel and careless beast...

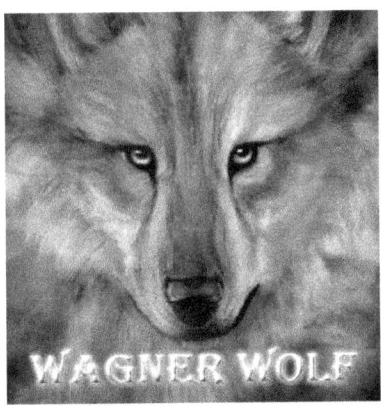

A Mother's Welcome

My dream was to become an interior designer. But when Erica came along, my dreams were not deferred, but changed. Her dreams became my dreams. Through her, I accomplished all the goals I could ever want in life.

She and I spent my adulthood trying to be thoughtful of others and to treat everyone fairly. I was comfortable sitting back in the wings and watching Erica, my precious daughter, rise to the top. I waited for her phone calls to ask me to help her do something, research, cut and paste projects, share thoughts or ideas.

But now she's not here and I intend to complete as many of her unfinished projects as I can. Her notes are very clear as to what direction she was headed. It's sort of like I'm filling in the blanks, and this finalized book is my love story to her...

[all entries written by Mrs. Josephine Holloman-Adams will be italicized to distinguish them from Erica's posts]

From The Author...

Hello, my name is Erica J. Holloman. I am a full-time doctoral student at the University of Louisville. Being here today is a testimony to God being real.

Finding my lump was purely by accident. I was not performing a self-breast exam. I wasn't looking for it, and wasn't sure what I had found. Being told at the age of 31 that you have cancer can be a difficult pill to swallow. I will never forget the day that I was diagnosed: October 2, 2007. My mother wanted to drive to Louisville to hear the results, but I wouldn't let her. In my heart I knew that the news wasn't going to be good. I compromised and let her listen on speaker phone because, like any mother, I knew she would have questions. When the doctor delivered the news, I cried softly so my mother wouldn't be able to hear through the phone. I gathered myself enough to let my mother know I would call her back.

I originally found the lump in August and knew then that I had cancer. I went beyond being afraid or assuming the worst, I knew. In a way, it kind of prepared me because I began dealing with it early. After leaving the doctor's office, I went to my car. There's no way to prepare yourself to hear the words, "You've got cancer." I called my mother on the phone and we cried. I allowed myself seven minutes to cry but would never again shed a tear over it. Strangely enough, on my diagnosis day I went to class. It was all I could do to hold it together, but I couldn't go home...alone...and be left to my thoughts.

The next couple of months were a whirlwind. I had a lumpectomy. My tumor was aggressive. I chose to fight. I chose to live. I have done everything I could possibly do to stay ahead of cancer. Even though that was the case, I delayed chemotherapy to undergo fertility preservation since chemotherapy would most certainly render me sterile. Instead of radiation, I opted for a double mastectomy and reconstruction. To some that may be considered radical, but I researched my options very carefully before choosing that route. I had a high risk for recurrence and years down the line, I didn't want to be dealing with this again. I just think about where I would be today if my doctors had told me that I was too young to have breast cancer. If I had to leave you with anything, it's to take control of your health. If you have a gut feeling about something, don't turn away from it. Many doctors don't advocate for mammograms earlier than 40, but you can request one. The price you pay for a mammogram is not more costly than the price you may pay by not having one.

Erica J. Holloman

Table Of Contents

PART 1 – Discovery & Diagnosis (18)

Depression (200)

PART 2 – The Saga Continues (207)

PART 3 – The Fertility Files (217)

Was I Really Dreaming (271)

Fertility Revisited (275)

Updates (292)

Glossary (301)

17

Breast Cancer Chronicles

By Erica J. Holloman, PhD

Part 1:
Discovery & Diagnosis

10.02.07

...I Have Breast Cancer...

OCTOBER 2007

S	M	T	W	T	F	S
	1	2	3	4	5	6
7	8	9	10	11	12	13
14	15	16	17	18	19	20
21	22	23	24	25	26	27
28	29	30	31			

Medications mentioned: None

Treatments mentioned: None

I have breast cancer.
My diagnosis date: October 2, 2007.
I am thirty-one years old with no history of breast cancer in my family.

For some of you, the last three sentences will cause you to be concerned. Am I okay? No, but I will be. As a means to process and for self-therapy, I will be blogging my experience. I jotted some thoughts down after finding my lump. And while you may not have been with me from the beginning, the blog entries will take you back to the first moments. The moment that my life began to change.....

8.20.07 -- 8.29.07

Uncertain...

This originated as a poem, but really ended up being a series of thoughts.

	AUGUST 2007					
S	M	T	W	T	F	S
	1	2	3	4	5	6
7	8	9	10	11	12	13
14	15	16	17	18	19	20
21	22	23	24	25	26	27
28	29	30	31			

Medications mentioned: None

Treatments mentioned: Mammogram

The saga began in August...... I found a lump today. I wasn't looking for it, it just kinda made itself known. It was hard to be sure of what exactly it was so I became very familiar with myself as I searched for the true nature of this foreign mass. I was still unsure. I didn't have anyone I trusted to help me verify what I thought. Maybe it'll go way. I'm on my period and maybe my body is going through a temporary change. Yep, it'll go away.

Everyday, several times a day, I find myself feeling on my breast....the left one. It seems to have planted itself there and taken root. I won't admit it out loud, but I'm concerned but not yet worried. I'm going to make an appointment to see a doctor. It's been a week already. For some reason, I think it'll disappear. That's not my kind of luck though.

I went to the doctor. She was able to find the lump without me telling her its location. Worrisome. She can feel it too. Usually the touch of a woman's hand on my breast is not wanted, but I welcomed it. She said I have to get a mammogram and an ultrasound. I'm 31. No history of breast cancer in my family. I don't smoke. I don't drink. I don't do drugs. I am not obese. Why me? I bet everyone asks that. It's a valid question. It's probably my caffeine addition. Who knew that Coca-Cola would be the cause of my demise?

My first mammogram. Not scary. Not painful. Just exposed. It's different when you take off your clothes because you choose to be intimate with someone. I can imagine that every woman feels uncomfortable at least once while wearing the notorious front-open robe. There is nothing like having your breasts manhandled by some stranger......but at least her hands were warm.

I can't say that the ultrasound was any better. I got a technician who was new on the job. To add insult to injury, I had to be the guinea pig. She attempted to do the ultrasound and then had to invite another person in to check her work. They stared together at the screen, but were unable to share the results with me. That's annoying as hell. I think it's cruel and unusual punishment to make someone wait damn near a week for results. It is truly impossible to concentrate 100% on any task with possible impending doom on your mind.

The verdict's in. I didn't quite get hit with a sledgehammer, but I have to get a biopsy. Suddenly, all of the small things that were bothering me that day didn't matter anymore.

> *Erica has a doctor's visit today. I want to go. She won't let me. Again she wins. I must respect her wishes as she reminds me that she is 31. I wait by the phone. She said she had to help the doctor find the spot. I think, 'good maybe it went away.' But she has more tests scheduled. I don't think, I just say "okay".*

"Reframe." I had to put my life in perspective. If nothing else, this would be a wake-up call. Life is really short. How do I want to live it? Life doesn't stop though. I still have to do my reading and homework assignments. I still have to fulfill the requirements of my internship. I am still going to get my Ph.D.

I still suffer in silence, though. Hiding the fact that I'm worried from most people. Wearing a smile for all to see while masking my fear. I am scared. I won't let it overtake me. I will do my best to remain optimistic because truth is.....I don't know anything yet. They can't tell me anything worse than what I've already thought. What if I have a tumor*? What if I have cancer*? What if I have to have chemotherapy? What if I lose all my hair? What if I have to have my breast removed? What if I die....

Lord, I pray that it is not in the plan for me to have breast cancer. I ask You that no matter what the outcome, You will walk with me. What doesn't kill me will make me stronger, I know...

9.24.07

Consultation

S	M	T	W	T	F	S
	1	2	3	4	5	6
7	8	9	10	11	12	13
14	15	16	17	18	19	20
21	22	23	24	25	26	27
28	29	30	31			

SEPTEMBER 2007

Medications: None

Treatments: Ultrasound guided needle biopsy

I was calm walking into the office. I was referred to this doctor by Student Health Services (SHS), so I was hoping she would be okay. SHS hadn't told me anything at all about how to prepare for this visit. Originally, I thought I would be having my biopsy on this day until I called the office myself to ask a question.

The doctor came in and had me lie down with my arm behind my head. During the examination, she was unable to find the lump. I had to place her hand on what I thought was the lump. She acknowledged that there could be something there and then ordered an ultrasound guided needle biopsy to help determine what exactly was going on.

I set my appointment for Thursday. I'm not excited about the prospect of getting this biopsy. I don't like needles. I don't like blood and I know both are going to be present on that day. Unfortunately, it is a necessary evil in this process.

9.27.07

Biopsy Part 1

	SEPTEMBER 2007					
S	M	T	W	T	F	S
	1	2	3	4	5	6
7	8	9	10	11	12	13
14	15	16	17	18	19	20
21	22	23	24	25	26	27
28	29	30	31			

Medications: None

Treatments: Biopsy

Thursday is the beginning of my weekend, so I thought it would give me some time to recover. After finding out that I had to have this biopsy, I told my mother what the doctor said. For some reason, she thought that she was going to come down to Louisville and be by my side. It was an outpatient procedure and she didn't need to be present for it. We debated about that for a while. I know that she's my mother and that's all she knows to do, but this was not a big deal.

I get to the hospital and they direct me to a triage area. There are all kinds of folks in here. It looked more like the outpatients recovery area where you see people laying in beds trying to wake up enough to go home. The nurse seats me in a 5 by 5 box (room) with at 19" plasma TV on the wall. I guess that was supposed to keep me entertained while I waited.

I pulled a book out of my bag. I was trying to study for my comprehensive exams, so I needed to utilize every possible moment I had to sneak in a read. All the while, orderlies are rolling patients in and out of the triage or to and from surgery.

The next thing I hear is this woman cry out in pain. She was screaming as loud as she could that she was in pain and that she has Multiple Sclerosis (MS). Nurses and orderlies kept walking past her as if she had said nothing at all. Seriously, I was mortified. I wanted to get up and help her. Finally, a nurse went to talk with her and then called her doctor to get her more drugs. I felt really sorry for her. The nurse helping me should've been helping her....I wasn't suffering.

> *Today, Erica is having an ultrasound-guided needle biopsy. I want to be there but she insists that I stay home. She's not being fair to me; my heart is aching on the inside. I'm sad but don't show it. I wait for the phone to ring just to hear her voice and to know she's okay.*

The nurse asked me all kinds of questions about my health. I answered and continued to wait. She told me that the radiologist who was performing my biopsy would be coming over to speak with me and explain the procedure. The radiologist was a short, bald, black man. He gave his spiel and then asked if I had any questions. I had to tell him that I didn't like needles or blood, especially my own blood. The last thing he wanted me to do was barf on his clothes.

I was then led to another room. It appeared to be the mammography waiting room. The nurse told me to disrobe from the waist up and put on the infamous "gown" that opens in the front. They were kind enough to provide me with a basket to put my clothes and personal effects in. After a few minutes, I was retrieved for my biopsy.

9.27.07

Biopsy Part 2

	SEPTEMBER 2007					
S	M	T	W	T	F	S
	1	2	3	4	5	6
7	8	9	10	11	12	13
14	15	16	17	18	19	20
21	22	23	24	25	26	27
28	29	30	31			

Medications: Local anesthesia

Treatments: Biopsy, x-ray

So, here I am lounging on this hospital bed. Lefty (my new name for my left breast) is once again being exposed to the elements. Luckily, Righty was able to remain in hiding. It's impossible to be modest. When I looked to my left, I saw my chest x-rays. I could visibly see the mass in question. It was bright white. To my right was the ultrasound machine.

The biopsy was an ultrasound-guided needle biopsy. I don't do needles or blood! The nurse gave me a towel to put over my face so I wouldn't have to witness the horror. I received local anesthesia. Surprisingly enough, the needle that they jammed into my breast wasn't painful. That first shot pretty much numbed the entire left side of my body. The radiologist hit me with two more shots though.

And the cutting began...during the procedure I could feel some pressure from the device he was using. Once he found the exact spot, he inserted something that would take a sample from the mass. It made this awful clicking sound. He said that he would remove as much as he could, but since it was against my chest wall, he may not be able to remove much.

The radiologist said that there was another area that caused him concern and he asked me if he could biopsy that area as well. I told him to do whatever he had to do while he was in there.

The procedure was over fairly quickly. After all that slicing and dicing meant cleanup was in order. The nurse prematurely removed the towel from my face. Even though I didn't see the blood, I'm aware that she was cleaning it up. I'm a bleeder! She applied some Derma-bond as the final touch and bandaged me up.

Talking to the radiologist afterward gave me great cause for concern. It was the words he chose and the tone. He merely confirmed what I had been thinking for some time. It wasn't good......

10.02.07

Diagnosis Day

	OCTOBER 2007					
S	M	T	W	T	F	S
	1	2	3	4	5	6
7	8	9	10	11	12	13
14	15	16	17	18	19	20
21	22	23	24	25	26	27
28	29	30	31			

Medications: None

Treatments: Lumpectomy, mastectomy

I walked into the doctor's office determined to be ready to hear whatever she had to throw at me. My mother so wanted to be present, but I managed to convince her to stay at home. We had argued for several days but my gut told me that she didn't need to be there. If the news was bad, I feared that she wouldn't be able to give me a kiss and a hug and then get back on the road like she said she would. No mother is going to leave her child following that kind of news. She was going to want to take care of me and I was going to want to take care of her, but life goes on. I was not going to have time to weep until after class was over later that day. It was better that she stayed home. My entire family was telling my mother that she needed to be there, she wanted to be there, but my wishes won out in the end.

But I did compromise. I let her listen to the diagnosis via telephone. The doctor began to speak and her tone from the beginning was grim. She didn't mince words. I was fine for the first few minutes of her explanation, but it really hit me when I began to think about how this was going to affect my class work. Being a full-time student is paying the bills right now. What was I going to do if I had to stop? I've been in school for 30 years and I don't know how not to be a student. My whole existence was in the balance.

I began to weep silently. I didn't want my mother to hear. The doctor handed me a box of tissues while she continued to explain the findings. I got it back together enough to ask my mother is she had any more questions. I told her that I would call her back in a few minutes. The doctor wanted me to make a decision between a lumpectomy and mastectomy in the next couple of days and then call back to schedule whichever procedure I chose.

The doctor left me to myself for a few minutes. I managed to recover some and then went out to schedule my appointment. My decision had been made....lumpectomy. I went out to the desk and they escorted me to another desk. In reflection, I kind of giggled to myself. The nurses kept offering me Coca-Cola as a soother. I declined. One nurse brought me a bag with a blanket in it. The pink blanket was from the Blanket of Hope Society.

I schedule my appointment for October 16. I made it to the car and then called my mother. I just started bawling. She was worried about me. When she heard me crying, she started crying too. It took me a few minutes to get my emotions under control and then I was okay again. I drove home and just sat there. I managed to make it to class that night. It was difficult. I told my professor. Needless to say, she was shocked. The words were still fresh. I had not finished processing them and here I am sharing with someone else. . I normally keep things to myself, but I realized I wouldn't be able to keep this from people. I was going to need help with this one.

I am sick with worry because she won't let me come to Louisville and go to the doctor's visit with her. I felt it wasn't good news and I wanted to be there. She agreed to let me call and listen while she was getting the results from the biopsy. The doctor introduced herself and wasted no time in telling us that Erica has breast cancer. I listened to the doctor talk. We both asked questions and then the phone was silent. I could tell she was crying. I wanted to cry.......

10.04.07

One Moment, Two Thoughts

	OCTOBER 2007					
S	M	T	W	T	F	S
	1	2	3	4	5	6
7	8	9	10	11	12	13
14	15	16	17	18	19	20
21	22	23	24	25	26	27
28	29	30	31			

Medications: None

Treatments: Chemotherapy

I cried myself to sleep last night. After being stoic all day, I was able to take a moment and give in to my weakness. Is it healthy to feel sorry for yourself? I harbor anxiety about my uncertain future.

I don't look forward to chemotherapy. I'm hoping that's not part of my future. I really don't want to lose my hair, although there are some really good wigs out there. When someone mentioned losing hair, I only thought about the hair on my head. I never thought about eyebrows, eyelashes, arm hair, leg hair, etc. I could do without the armpit and/or leg hair though.

10.05.07 -- 10.07.07

My Trip To The ER

	October 2007					
S	M	T	W	T	F	S
	1	2	3	4	5	6
7	8	9	10	11	12	13
14	15	16	17	18	19	20
21	22	23	24	25	26	27
28	29	30	31			

Medications: None

Treatments: Visit to Emergency Room

For the last few days I've noticed the hole in my breast (the biopsied area) slowly turning red. The Derma-bond is still intact, so I wasn't sure what was going on. I could see the blood rising to the top of the wound. Finally the blood began to spill out of the wound. I decided to watch it one more day to determine whether it was something to be concerned about.

I got back from the Circle City Classic in Indianapolis. The blood was coming out even more and I felt nauseous. That could've been due to my reluctance to look at my own blood, though. I let my mother look at the area to see what she thought. I decided to call the Radiology department at the hospital that performed my biopsy. I described what I saw and how I was feeling and they told me to wait until tomorrow and call the breast care nurse. Considering the way that I was feeling, I wasn't going to wait until the next day. Hell, I thought I might have ripped open the incision or have internal bleeding.

My mom decided to call Ask-a-Nurse to see if she could get some information. I gave the nurse all of the pertinent information and she recommended that I visit an Urgent Care or an Emergency Room (ER) within the next 3 hours! This woman had me believing that I was about to die. It was like she gave me a deadline to live! I considered going to Urgent Care and thought better of it. I decided to go to the ER at Jewish Kenwood because I thought it would have the least traffic. Service was quick. I was only sitting in the waiting room for three minutes before the nurse called me back. I've noticed from this ordeal that it is very difficult for me to be modest. I can't tell you the number of people who I've been 'exposed' to in the last few weeks.

I got a male doctor this time He looked at what was going on and determined that is was a hematoma. He peeled all of the Derma-bond off and scraped of the excess skin, blood, and pus leaving a gaping hole in my breast. Okay, maybe that's an exaggeration, but there really is a gaping hole there. He assured me that a hematoma wasn't a big deal and that the nurse would just throw a band-aid on there and everything would be fine. We waited for the nurse to come but instead another doctor came in. He claimed that he wanted to check the hole in my chest. But he really had no apparent reason to be there. The previous doctor mentioned that he thought my mother was attractive. It was clear to me that this doctor wasn't really interested in seeing this hole in my chest, but wanted to get a peek at my mother. What I can't figure out is why I have to bare my breast to accomplish this! I felt used. The nurse finally came in and bandaged me up and it was time to go.

10.15.07

Thoughts Before My Surgery

	October 2007					
S	M	T	W	T	F	S
	1	2	3	4	5	6
7	8	9	10	11	12	13
14	15	16	17	18	19	20
21	22	23	24	25	26	27
28	29	30	31			

Medications: None

Treatments: None

I attended the "Making Strides Cancer Walk" yesterday. I went this time in a new capacity...a Survivor. In previous years, I have volunteered my time helping to celebrate those who have survived this ordeal and give a moment of thought to those who weren't so fortunate.

It just felt so different. I brought Kisha and Shannon with me to the walk. They wanted to share the experience with me and show their support. I walked into the Survivor tent and walked up to the table. The volunteer asked if I was a Survivor. I paused for a moment and then I said, "yes." Acceptance. She smiled and then said that i needed a hat. All survivors wore pink caps that day. I walked further down the table and another volunteer asked if I had gotten a lei. I had not and she quickly got up and got a lei for me and put it around my neck. She hugged me and gave me some positive words.

Today, I am hopeful. I am nervous and anxious. My body is having a different reaction than my mind. My body tells me that I am stressed. My head tells me that I am stressed because it hurts. My mind tells me that I am ready to go get this over with. Tomorrow, I will go to sleep and then wake up with the evil mass removed from my body. I hope they get it all. I don't want to go through this again. I'm about to go eat a snack because all food gets cut off at midnight. I'll see you all on the other side of cancer!

10.16.07

Surgery Day

S	M	T	W	T	F	S
	1	2	3	4	5	6
7	8	9	10	11	12	13
14	15	16	17	18	19	20
21	22	23	24	25	26	27
28	29	30	31			

October 2007

Medications: Lidocaine, Anesthetics

Treatments: IV placement, Lumpectomy, Chemo

My mother came back to Louisville with me the night before my surgery. Some of my family and extended family came down the morning of my surgery. As with any surgery, the patient is not allowed to eat anything after midnight. I woke up starving. I had to report to the hospital at 11:30 a.m. That is an incredibly long time to be without food. My so-called 'family' gets to my house at 9:00 a.m. and proceeds to eat breakfast right in front of me. I'm talking eggs, bacon, biscuits, and fruit. My feelings were hurt!

The phones started ringing off the hook because people knew we were leaving the house at 11:00 a.m. My pastor called and he prayed with me. We left my apartment at 11:00 a.m. with two carloads of people. There were lots of people in the waiting room. All I walked in with was a pair of warm fuzzy socks. I handed everything else to my mom and we went and sat down.

Two minutes later, the nurse was calling my name. It was time. I told my family that I loved them and followed the nurse. She took me back to a small room with a stretcher. She gave me a gown and told me to get totally undressed. I still don't understand why removing my panties was a necessity, but that is neither here nor there.

Nurses were shuffling themselves in and out of the tiny space. One nurse marked my breast. She wrote the word "correct" above my breast to make sure the doctors were not going to operate on the wrong one. I let her know that I appreciated that. Another nurse made sure I was warm enough and added layers of warm blankets. And another nurse connected my IV.

Now let me say a few words about this damn IV. I always tell nurses that I don't want the IV in my hand because that crap hurts like hell. She decides that she wants to put it in my hand but insists that she can numb it sufficiently enough that it won't hurt. I'm thinking she's gonna rub the Lidocaine on my hand to numb it, but she gets a needle out and shoots my hand with it!

> *Two car loads of family members came down this morning. I know Erica can't eat but what am I supposed to tell them?!*

Part of this lumpectomy was having a sentinel node biopsy. This involved shooting a blue dye into my skin that would go to the lymph nodes. They would remove this lymph node and send it down to pathology during the procedure to determine whether any cancer had spread to any other lymph nodes. I had to go down to Radiology about forty-five minutes prior to the procedure to get the blue dye. Earlier the nurses tried to prepare me for the procedure by putting Lidocaine on my breast. This was 'supposed' to help numb the area. Let me be the first to say..."that shit did not help!" Excuse my language, but this procedure is real messed up.

The radiologist started putting the damn dye in and it felt like someone was sticking a straight pin into my breast. He must've stuck me like four or five times. They told me I did well because I did not cry or scream. They said that most women can be heard screaming from the hallway. I will say it hurt like hell and I won't say anymore about it.

They rolled me back upstairs and let my family come in to see me prior to leaving for surgery. They could only come back in pairs and my mother and grandmother came back first and then my aunt. The pastor had told my grandmother not to let me go into surgery without someone praying over me, so my aunt called her husband so he could pray via telephone. Then my grandmother put her hand over my forehand (or was it her forehead?) and started saying some words. When she did that, I started to cry. I was scared.

> It seemed to be a long wait. When they finally told me I could come back to see her, my mom came with me. I stayed a few minutes just to see her face, then I left to allow the others to have a chance to see her – they took too long. I went back in with her. The time had come for her to go to surgery and it was the first time that Erica said that she was scared. I told her that I was scared too. She started to cry. And as I looked into her eyes, I started to cry too. We both finally admitted it - we were scared.

> The crying only lasted a few minutes because as the others came in, we popped back into "strong" mode and stopped crying. Never let them see you cry. As they wheeled her away, I, her mother was allowing the life of my daughter to be in the hands of someone else. I could not help her. I was suffering silently, just waiting, standing still.

They must have started the anesthesia drip before they wheeled me downstairs. I remember making it to the surgical area and seeing the doctor, but then it was lights out after that.

> The doctor came out and got me and my husband to give us the results of the surgery. She took us to a small room just large enough for her to sit across from us. The artwork on the walls was your typical hospital pictures, maybe flowers. She told us that it took long because at first they could not find the spot where the lump was, so they had to give her another ultrasound and then do the surgery. She told us the stage that the cancer was at, the size, etc. She

said she was worried about Erica because she was the strong silent type and you cannot be sure how patients like her will handle the situation. Then she said that Erica would have to have chemotherapy and radiation. We thanked her and left to tell the family. For the first time, I cried in front of my family. How was I supposed to tell her that the one thing she said she did not want, was what she had to have? CHEMO.

I remember slightly coming to and dry heaving. My body does not like anesthesia, it wanted it out. I remember my mother talking to me and asking if I wanted some ice chips. I don't remember saying, "yes" but I do so remember her saying quite a few time that I need to wake up and swallow the ice chips. I kept falling asleep with them in my mouth.

I remember waking up again with dry heaves. I kept trying to say that I had to pee. The words would not form correctly. They managed to understand me. They were preparing me to go to the bathroom when the unthinkable happened. I peed on myself while dry heaving. Then I managed to pee and vomit at the same time and then I felt fine. My mother and aunt were good sports because they had to clean me up.

> *I wanted them to keep her in the hospital overnight, but they said that they were going to let her go home. Little did I know that the heifer was going to pee on me! She tried to tell us but couldn't. Then ya'll....I had to clean it up!*

I remember getting into the wheelchair, sort of rolling down the hallway to the hospital entrance and getting in the car. For some reason, my mother kept asking me questions and apparently, I was mumbling incoherent things. I think that she was just entertaining herself.

> *I wanted them to keep her, but no. She was alert enough to give directions to her house. All she wanted to know was, "What did the doctor say" and "Do I have to have chemo?" The first time she asked we were sitting in the car outside the hospital. We were all silent. Someone asked, "Which way do we go?" She gave directions. The next time she asked what the doctor said, her tone was*

demanding. I said we would talk when we go home. She was argumentative. She asked again as soon as we got into the house. Everyone scattered, leaving me to tell her. She was angry. "Why didn't you just tell me?" she said. I didn't know how or when would be the right time.

10.19.07

The Oncologist

Treatment, Fertility, And Hair...Oh My!

	OCTOBER 2007					
S	M	T	W	T	F	S
	1	2	3	4	5	6
7	8	9	10	11	12	13
14	15	16	17	18	19	20
21	22	23	24	25	26	27
28	29	30	31			

Medications: None

Treatments: Chemo, Radiation, Social Worker visit

I scheduled to see the oncologist shortly after my surgery because I need to get the ball rolling. I needed to see the oncologist before I saw a fertility specialist. On this day, I had to do some initial blood work, following which I met with a social worker. My mother was with me for this appointment. We were taken to the office of the social worker and waited for her to arrive.

The social worker seemed to be a nice woman, but I don't know what she expected. Yes, I am young. Yes, I live in this city without family. Yes, getting cancer sucks, but I've made peace with cancer. She would ask me questions and I would answer them and then there would be these incredibly long pauses. It was very awkward. I think she was trying to analyze me, but she won't figure me out.

> *The social worker's office was cozy and she was nice. I know that having cancer stinks, but the way she spoke was all doom and gloom. Erica keeps looking at me and I keep looking at her making faces. Maybe we are not normal. I kicked her foot because the*

> social worker would make long pauses. What was she waiting for....crying, depression, sorrow? I'm thinking, "Can you get us some money or not," because this other stuff - we got this!

After meeting with her, it was time to meet with the oncologist. I'm not sure what I expected. He was more stuffy than I expected. He came in pretty much with a course of treatment. He explained things to me as if I was six years old. He repeated himself a lot. Finally, I told him that I was ready to get this party started, so let's do it.

He let me know that all of the cancer had been removed. He also said that due to my age he thought it was best to be as aggressive as possible, so I wouldn't have to do this again down the line. He thought chemotherapy was the next option and then radiation. I originally thought I would be able to get away without chemo. I hadn't really prepared to hear it from the doctor although my mother told me that the surgeon believed that I would need it. I had to re-verify with him that hair loss would be a reality with chemo. He wasn't very sensitive on this issue.

61

What can a woman expect from a male oncologist anyway?

I told him that one of my biggest concerns was fertility issues. Someday, I'd like to be able to have children. He referred me to the best fertility specialist in Louisville. I will need to have my eggs harvested prior to chemo. The timeline is tight, since chemo needs to start soon.

10.19.07

The Next Few Days

	OCTOBER 2007					
S	M	T	W	T	F	S
	1	2	3	4	5	6
7	8	9	10	11	12	13
14	15	16	17	18	19	20
21	22	23	24	25	26	27
28	29	30	31			

Medications: None

Treatments: None

I am really alone these days. My Mother has been my constant companion. She's been there for me when I couldn't be there for myself. I need her more now than I've ever needed her. She gets on my nerves sometimes, but that's an undocumented part of the job description.

Other than nausea, I've only noticed a loss of pubic hair. And who's complaining about that? Not me!!! I wish I could shave it this smooth. This is Awesome. I knew there had to be some perk to this mess. WhooHoo!!

10.21.07

Hair, Oh Hair!

	October 2007					
S	M	T	W	T	F	S
	1	2	3	4	5	6
7	8	9	10	11	12	13
14	15	16	17	18	19	20
21	22	23	24	25	26	27
28	29	30	31			

Medications: None

Treatments: Chemotherapy

Well, with chemotherapy there's hair loss. This has been a hard one to wrap my mind around. I'm not claiming to be like Samson in the Bible, but hair is a permanent accessory. For those who know me well, they know that I get my relaxer every six weeks like clockwork. I like my hair bone straight. I will admit that I look good with a short cut, but with a short, short cut? I was talking with another survivor who happens to be a hairdresser. She cut all of her hair off - I mean she went bald prior to chemo. I asked her if she did that to save herself the trauma of watching her hair fall out. She said, "yes."

On the bright side, no hair saves a lot of money at the hairdresser. On the other side, my hair has been a great part of my existence. I am sad to part with it, but am hopeful that it will grow back straight as some people have indicated. I look forward to a hair texture change or it could grow back in a different color. The hairdresser said that she's going to make me a wig at no cost. For that, I am grateful. I'm sure it will be nice.

> It's ironic that one day I saw a little black girl with cancer that needed a wig. The wig would be from human hair to fit her head and would cost a lot of money. But if people donated their hair, children like her could get the wigs for free. Since then, I have donated my hair three times. When the oncologist told Erica that she would probably lose her hair, I had no words to say because I knew that I could not give her my hair...no words.

So, my mother got mad because I told her that I don't want anyone to ask to see my head once my hair is gone. The situation is traumatic enough. I also told her that I don't want to be in any Thanksgiving, Christmas, or birthday pictures. Then she had the nerve to tell me that it's not fair. I told her that she didn't want to talk about fair and then I just started bawling. I had to get off the phone. That'll be the end of that conversation.

10.23.07

What Am I Going To Do About Class?

	OCTOBER 2007					
S	M	T	W	T	F	S
	1	2	3	4	5	6
7	8	9	10	11	12	13
14	15	16	17	18	19	20
21	22	23	24	25	26	27
28	29	30	31			

Medications: None

Treatments: Chemotherapy

On top of everything else, the flu hits me. I thought that I was going to be able to start my week today, but that is dead in the water. I had set an appointment with my advisor to discuss issues with class, but we had to do that over the telephone because a sista got chills right now.

I felt a little better after speaking with my advisor. I was worried about getting behind in class work. I will probably take a few incompletes for my coursework because there's no way I can keep up now. My mind really is scattered. I'll be two weeks behind at this point and with chemo starting in the near future, who knows how my body will react.

10.24.2007

I'm A Survivor

	OCTOBER 2007					
S	M	T	W	T	F	S
	1	2	3	4	5	6
7	8	9	10	11	12	13
14	15	16	17	18	19	20
21	22	23	24	25	26	27
28	29	30	31			

Medications: None

Treatments: Chemotherapy, Radiation, Lumpectomy

The following words will probably come as a shock to many of you who read this. Before I say anything else....I am okay.

I have breast cancer. I am 31 years old. Breast cancer does not run in my family! My diagnosis date was October 2, 2007. It is a date that will be forever seared into my memory. I had a lumpectomy on October 16, 2007. All of the cancer is believed to have been removed, but for safety precautions, I will be undergoing chemotherapy and radiation.

Once the diagnosis has been made, things move at a pretty quick pace. Many decisions have to be made (continue classes vs. discontinue, lumpectomy vs. mastectomy, fertility issues, chemo, etc.). I am still in the process of making decisions. I am emotionally and physically fatigued as you can probably imagine.

My biggest challenge has been monetary. For those of you who have Student Health Insurance, we all know that it doesn't cover much. But I have a wonderful family who have started a raffle at home in Cincinnati to raise funds.

For those of you wondering whether I will be continuing classes, the answer is, "hopefully." I will probably start chemo towards the end of November. Professors have been wonderful with flexibility. Most likely, I will have to take an "I" in my classes. Fortunately, this was my last semester of class work prior to writing my dissertation, so it won't be a setback.

For those of you in Louisville, I will be around...some. I'll be sporting a new 'do' courtesy of chemotherapy. Life will continue for me. It's important to put things in perspective...I'm not in a crashing airplane...I haven't lost any of my senses...and I still got my mama. I am okay. There will be six months of trying times, but I will make it through.

Breast cancer wasn't supposed to find me or so I thought. What you read out there suggests that breast cancer is more prevalent in families with a history of breast cancer. 80% of women with breast cancer DID NOT have a family history of it. That means that each one of you needs to do monthly self-breast exams. I will admit to not regularly doing self-exams. I located my mass by accident. It was not in the fatty tissue of the breast but up high on my chest wall.

Luckily, I was familiar enough to know that something was not right. My breast cancer was caught in Stage 1 (early), but it was Grade 4 (fast growing). If I had waited another few weeks, I could be having an entirely different experience. I say these things not to scare any of you, but to convince you to save your own life!

Let it be said that men can also get breast cancer. Men you also need to do self-breast exams. It is not embarrassing! Anyone who produces estrogen can get breast cancer, which means men and women.

Please do not feel sorry for me. I am blessed. Many have survived BC. I will be added to the list. If you see me, it's okay to ask how I'm doing. I'll probably give you the standard line, "I'm good," and we'll both keep rolling.

I want to thank the people who have been praying for me and sending positive energy my way. If I call you my friend that means I love you. 1 in 8 women will get breast cancer. I share these words to save a life.

11.01.07

The Struggle For Motherhood

		NOVEMBER 2007				
S	M	T	W	T	F	S
				1	2	3
4	5	6	7	8	9	10
11	12	13	14	15	16	17
18	19	20	21	22	23	24
25	26	27	28	29	30	

Medications: None

Treatments: Fertility Options

I went to the fertility specialist today. He did not provide me with any news that I wanted to hear. He gave me five fertility options. Whichever I choose, it has to be soon because things have to be done prior to receiving chemotherapy.

Option 1: Egg Donor
This is where some other woman provides an egg and my future partner would fertilize the egg. The baby would be half of him and none of me. For a known egg donor, this can cost up to $16,000. Usually, this would be a sister, but I'm an only child. My cousin agreed to donate, but she's 36 -- too old by industry standards. Egg donors usually fall between 20-32 years old. The process is more expensive for an anonymous donor because you have to pay that person and the cost starts at $23,000.

Option 2: In-vitro Maturation
In this process, they take my immature eggs, mature them in the lab and then fertilize them with donor sperm. Prior to speaking with the fertility specialist, I thought I would be able to provide my own donor, but I was quickly informed that would not be possible. Sperm donations have

to be tested, frozen and quarantined for 180 days to make sure the specimen is not carrying any diseases. Fresh sperm is out of the question. What's been difficult for me is the notion of a stranger fertilizing my egg. This costs between $2,000 and $4,000 depending on how far along I would get in the process. The number above does not include the price of embryo storage.

Option 3: Egg Freezing
This process involves over-stimulating the ovaries to produce eggs to be extracted. This isn't a good option because I will produce estrogen, and producing estrogen can help cancer grow. Not to mention that you have to give yourself daily injections for 10-12 days and I don't do needles! Plus, this is experimental.

Option 4: Chemo-protection
This involved shutting down production in my ovaries with drugs. Chemotherapy attacks growing cells, so if my ovaries are shut down, theoretically this will help shield my eggs from the effects of chemo. This is also experimental and costs between $5,000 and $6,000.

Option 5: No Treatment
Just take my chances and hope my ovaries work and that I come out of menopause following chemotherapy. Miracles required here.

Today was a bad one. My hopes of motherhood seem bleak. I wanted to have two kids by twenty-three. My mother had me at seventeen and I wanted to replicate the closeness of our relationship by having kids young. I told myself that I would not have children after thirty. Now here I am....thirty-one years old with no kids, with cancer, and hopes of bearing a child -- fleeting.

I've always wanted to be a mother and I've never wanted to be a mother. I know that sounds weird, but choosing to become a mother is one of the biggest decisions a woman will make in her life. Letting go of all of your selfishness and unconditionally loving another is not the easiest thing to do. I often doubt my maternal instincts, but I've played mama to many young people. Taking care of people comes naturally for me. I resent that I have to make these decisions. I shouldn't have to.

I'm angry. Today was the first time I seriously thought, "Why me?" I have been a trooper through this whole process, but the fertility specialist gave me a reality check. I don't ever remember feeling so low. Then I realized that for the first time in my life.....

I'm depressed. At times, I feel like I'm being punished. I tried to live the best way I know how. I wanted to wait until I got married before having children. My choices are not mine anymore. A hard lesson to learn is that you are not really in control.

I'm hard-headed. I'm going to need a divine intervention on this one. I will not choose Option 1, because the baby won't be biologically part of me. It is important to me that this baby be half of me, not half of whomever and some other woman. I might as well adopt a baby. It would be cheaper. Option 3, can't really be a consideration because producing estrogen is dangerous for my body at this point. I wouldn't seriously consider Option 5 because God made technology for a reason. I can do something and even if it doesn't work out, I will have made some effort.

I don't know yet which option(s) I will choose. The doctor gave me a website to look for sperm donors. I go back to the fertility specialist on Thursday. I have to have an answer for him because time is precious.

11.07.07

Wonder Woman

		NOVEMBER 2007				
S	M	T	W	T	F	S
				1	2	3
4	5	6	7	8	9	10
11	12	13	14	15	16	17
18	19	20	21	22	23	24
25	26	27	28	29	30	

Medications: None

Treatments: None

This ordeal has been interesting. I've had the opportunity to see myself through the eyes of others. For some reason, people believe I'm this strong woman. I often wonder who they are talking about. They couldn't possibly be talking about me. Most days I feel like that couldn't be further from the truth.

I don't know this woman they're talking about. Who is she? Where is she? It's all a facade. I'm not the woman they think I am. If I tried to write a list of strong women I knew, I wouldn't land on my own list. I just don't think of myself that way. I sometimes compare myself to Mr. Spock (or any other Vulcan). I spend most of my time not feeling anything - it's safer that way.

I am on emotion overload. It's like I don't know what to do with these continual waves of anger. My system has never had to deal with this amount of emotion at once and quite frankly it has left me stressed and fatigued.

11.02.07 – 11.08.07

Looking For My Baby's Daddy

	NOVEMBER 2007					
S	M	T	W	T	F	S
				1	2	3
4	5	6	7	8	9	10
11	12	13	14	15	16	17
18	19	20	21	22	23	24
25	26	27	28	29	30	

Medications: None

Treatments: Cryo Bank Visit

After about 24 hours of milling it over and a good night's sleep, I settled into my choices and chose Option 2 (in-vitro maturation) in combination with Option 4 (chemo-protection). While that day in particular was bad, I woke up the next day with the answer as clear as the sky.

I visited the cryobank that my doctor recommended. In my mind, I kinda turned the search into a game. Ya'll don't know how disgusted I was at first at the thought of this, so I made considerable improvements in one day's time.

Anyway, I had to determine my search criteria. My natural preference is Black men. Other than that, the only other criterion I used was height, 5'10" - 6'4". If I have a son, I wanted to give him a chance because short genes run rampant in my family. That search yielded only six men.

I spoke with some folks and decided to broaden my horizons a bit and change the selection criteria. I opened the search to bi-racial or multi-racial men. So now I have thirty-four more to consider. Keep in mind that this encompasses a racial/ethnic backgrounds. I ran into ▇lians, Israelis, English, Asian, Irish, and ▇ can think of was mixed in there.

Since I'm light skinned, I decided to try to find someone with some color. Each donor completes a short essay about why they chose to donate their sperm. A staff member gives their opinion on how they perceive the person and their looks. Also, the donor fills out a short profile, which includes general demographic information and what kinds of hobbies, skills, or activities they are involved in.

I was having a difficult time making this decision alone, so I gathered me a team of people I trust to help. This process is not an easy one because you can only judge by their writing. So I found myself analyzing their handwriting and paying close attention to what they said and didn't say.

After narrowing the field down to four donors, I decided to order their long profiles. The long profile gives detailed demographic and health information on their parents, grandparents, aunts and uncles, and other relatives. This cryo bank is making tons of money because each profile was $16. You can order baby pics for $21 each or personality profiles for $16 each. Their racket is so good that you can even bundle it. I decided to take my chances and just order the long profile.

> *Thanks for allowing me in the search for your baby's daddy, because based on what I see in some of the information on these families' histories - how about no. Some of them are out of the question. After much reading and conversation, we all agreed on the same one. Hopefully, she won't need them.*

I'm glad I ordered these long profiles because some of these folks' families are jacked up. One guy's maternal side of the family were all alcoholics. Another, his paternal side all had heart issues or high blood pressure. Two guy's families had schizophrenics. Somebody else had liver disease. It was too much for me and as I leafed through the donors, the information just got worse.

There was one, however, that stood out...

Sample - sperm donor application

Math Skills/Ability: _Advanced math skills, participated in many competitions_
Mechanical Skills: _Construction (Foundation, Plumbing, electricity)_
Athletic Skills: _Middle school - Football, High school - Wrestling, Basketball, Cheerleading_

What is your favorite sport? _Football_
What languages do you speak? _English + Spanish_
Hobbies/Talents: _Computers, Music (play the piano, cello, and saxophone), Public Speaking, Volunteering, sports_
Describe your artistic abilities: _Photography and image editing_

What are your favorite foods? _Greek and Lebanese, Mexican, and Italian_

What is your favorite color? _Yellow_
Do you like animals? If so, which is your favorite? _Dogs, especially the Alaskian Husky (or Hoskie) and its cousin the Akita_
To where would you like to travel and why? _Everywhere, mainly Latin American countries. I have never been the one to stay home long, and I love to immerse myself in different cultures_
How would you describe your personality? _Outgoing, spontaneous, friendly, gentleman, active, self-motivating, energetic_

What is your ultimate ambition or goal in life? How do you see yourself in twenty years?
To become a physician and practise in a hospital, also find my eternal companion. In twenty years I see myself fully employed and lots of kids.

CCB-0001, 2/95   -2-   Donor #: **25**

11.08.07 – 11.25.07

And The Winner Is...

NOVEMBER 2007						
S	M	T	W	T	F	S
				1	2	3
4	5	6	7	8	9	10
11	12	13	14	15	16	17
18	19	20	21	22	23	24
25	26	27	28	29	30	

Medications: None

Treatments: Fertility Preservation

My future baby's daddy is number 2500. I think I'll name the baby 25 for short to pay homage to the anonymous sperm donor. Just jokes people!

I'm okay with the decision and I have to keep in mind that this is the last resort. Hopefully, my ovaries will be tough enough to stand chemo and will be fine.

Since my doctors know that fertility preservation is important to me, we collectively have decided to put chemo off for a few more weeks, since I had ovulated already by the time we started this process. The doctors hope to extract up to three eggs. I'm hoping they get at least one egg because if they don't then I just paid $500 for some sperm I can't even use.

11.17.07

Hair Today, Gone Tomorrow

S	M	T	W	T	F	S
				1	2	3
4	5	6	7	8	9	10
11	12	13	14	15	16	17
18	19	20	21	22	23	24
25	26	27	28	29	30	

November 2007

Medications: None

Treatments: Haircut

Some of you may have noticed that I cut my hair. This was actually the third cut in preparation for chemo and its side effects. I wanted to go bald but my mother wouldn't let me. Hell, cutting it this low would've been traumatic for my hairdresser. I had her cut my hair down to about 2.5" on top. I was trying to get my hair like Jacqui Reid's, but it didn't work. Seriously ya'll, my mom was calling me "rooster" and I just couldn't have that.

When my stepfather came home later that night, I told him that I was going to ask him to cut and shave my hair down to natural. Even though I still had some relaxed hair, I just planned on moussing it to see what happened. My hope was that it would curl up.

He went and got his clippers and we just chopped the rest of my hair off. My stepfather is not a barber and I was looking crazy. I did wash my hair and mousse it the next day. It curled up like I thought, but the hair was uneven and I needed some help to tame it. I had to call in some favors.

Two days later, I went to the stylist who made one of my wigs and she agreed to help get this hair under control. I wanted her to just shape it, but somehow she ended up putting a texturizer in my hair. She cut it...and cut it...and cut it down. It's about a half an inch long on the top. I had to grow into it, but I like it. I put a scarf on, go to sleep, wake up, and keep it moving. I love that it's easy to maintain.

Surprisingly, this hair cut has been liberating. I can't really describe in words the transformation that my mental state has gone through to get to this place. Breast cancer is still betting on getting me down, but this fight is not over!

12.01.07

On The Rocks
(The Fertility Clinic)

	DECEMBER 2007					
S	M	T	W	T	F	S
					1	
2	3	4	5	6	7	8
9	10	11	12	13	14	15
16	17	18	19	20	21	22
23	24	25	26	27	28	29
30	31					

Medications: General Anesthesia

Treatments: Egg Retrieval

Let me just say...it has been a tough week. These last ten days I have been dealing with fertility issues. As I mentioned before, having the option to be a mother in the future is important to me. I was assured that my doctor is the best in Louisville, so I'm pretty confident that this will work out. I've been taking medications to get my ovaries under control. Darn near every day I've been going into the office to get a vaginal ultrasound and a blood test. These tests would determine which days I was ovulating and when they would be able to extract my eggs.

Friday was the "big day." I had to have someone come to the hospital with me because of the general anesthesia. My mom and aunt came down. We arrived at the office pretty early. When the doctors came in prior to the procedure they came in with black rain clouds over their heads. They told me that my estradiol levels were very low. During a normal procedure they would retrieve between zero and three eggs. Today, it seemed like my luck would bring me zero.

They went over all the details for my mom and aunt. Even if they were able to retrieve any eggs, the eggs would still have to survive maturation and then be able to be fertilized and survive the freezing to be a viable embryo. The procedure was supposed to take forty-five minutes.

> *World, meet 'Fertile Myrtle'. She was really sleepy when they brought her back. The first question she asked was "did they get any eggs?". I explained, "They got 7 and you made history." She smiled and fell back to sleep. She woke up five minutes later and asked did they get any eggs. I laughed and had to explain five more times - "yes, they did".*

Two hours passed and I was brought back to my mini cubicle. Ten minutes earlier one of the doctors had come out to let my mother know that they had not only retrieved three eggs, but six eggs and possible seven! They underestimated ya girl! Never in the history of the office had they ever retrieved that many eggs. I made history ya'll! So much for that black cloud. They won't make the mistake of misinterpreting the next female's estradiol levels.

The next day, they informed me that two of the six eggs had matured (the 7th turned out to be a shell). They then fertilized the eggs and froze them. Finally, a total of four matured, but only three made it. I have three embryos on ice for later usage.

12.03.07

The Rough Week Continues... Et Tu, Brute?

December 2007

S	M	T	W	T	F	S
						1
2	3	4	5	6	7	8
9	10	11	12	13	14	15
16	17	18	19	20	21	22
23	24	25	26	27	28	29
30	31					

Medications: Antibiotics, Pain Medication, Lupron

Treatments: Mammogram, Ultrasound, Biopsy

After the surgery they put me on antibiotics and pain meds. My mom drove us back to Cincy immediately following the procedure because my aunt had to get home to take her shot. I pretty much slept for 36 hours. I had to get back to take my first Lupron* shot (chemo-protection) on Sunday. I got on the road at 6:30 a.m. to make it back to Louisville. I had to stop my pain meds early the night before so my mind would be clear enough to make it back. That was a rough drive.

Earlier in the week...I was a part of this chemotherapy clinical trial, and it was necessary for me to have a bilateral mammogram. So the research nurse scheduled a mammogram and an ultrasound. The results needed to come back fairly quickly because I start chemo on the 6th. Well, the results came back...

They saw something on the films, but only on one of them. I was scheduled to have another ultrasound at another hospital (why, I don't know). Long story short - I will be having another biopsy on my other breast ASAP. My body is turning against me for some reason.

No worries though. The decisions that need to be made have already been made (I've watched the Matrix too many times). To be continued....

12.10.07

Chemoville, Here I Come

December 2007						
S	M	T	W	T	F	S
						1
2	3	4	5	6	7	8
9	10	11	12	13	14	15
16	17	18	19	20	21	22
23	24	25	26	27	28	29
30	31					

Medications: Fluouracil, Epirubicin, Cytoxan

Treatments: Biopsy, Chemotherapy

The biopsy on the right breast was benign. So, I will be moving forward with chemo. I am participating in a clinical trial, which is comparing the American standard of chemo versus the European standard of chemo. I was randomized to six cycles of the European standard of chemotherapy...FEC (fluouracil, epirubicin, cytoxan).

My first treatment is on the fourteenth. How am I feeling about that? Nervous. I don't like to be nauseous, but I have been assured that they have medicines that can prevent that. We'll see....

12.13.07

Pay It Forward

	DECEMBER 2007					
S	M	T	W	T	F	S
						1
2	3	4	5	6	7	8
9	10	11	12	13	14	15
16	17	18	19	20	21	22
23	24	25	26	27	28	29
30	31					

Medications: None

Treatments: Lab work, Chemotherapy Preparation

Me and my mom drove down from Cincinnati to Louisville the day before chemotherapy for what is to be a standard appointment with the doctor. Each time I go they will draw some blood to make sure my red and white blood counts are okay.

> *Looking around the Oncology office, everyone in the waiting room is my age or older. I know they think it's me with cancer. I wish I could trade places with her, but it's not me and I cannot.*

While I was sitting in the waiting room of Consultants in Blood Disorders & Cancer, I noticed that I was the youngest in the room. The average age in that room had to be sixty-five. I felt out of place.

Two nurses from the research department came out to see me. We talked for a few moments about what the next day's process would be and my mom had an opportunity to put faces with names of people that she had been hearing about. After they left, I went back to reading my book. Right after they left, a woman walked up to me and placed a sticky note on the book I was reading. She told me to call her anytime if I wanted to talk. She quickly told me that she overheard the nurses speaking to me and that she had been diagnosed with Hodgkin's lymphoma eight years ago. She thought I looked about her age when she was diagnosed and asked how old I was. I told her and she said that everything would be fine. The nurse called her name and she left. Her name was Donna. I was amazed at the pure generosity of this woman. To share a bit of herself and her story with me...I have to remember to pay it forward.

12.15.07

Chemo Day

			DECEMBER 2007			
S	M	T	W	T	F	S
					1	
2	3	4	5	6	7	8
9	10	11	12	13	14	15
16	17	18	19	20	21	22
23	24	25	26	27	28	29
30	31					

Medications: Anti-emetics, FEC

Treatments: Chemotherapy

My appointment was at 10:30AM. I drove to the CBC, but I was careful to make sure my mother had the directions because she would be driving back. Upon arriving, I checked in at the front desk and was given an arm bracelet. I was then directed back to the chemo area where I had to sign in and sit in a small waiting room.

There were about three people in front of me, but my wait wasn't too long. I told the nurse I'd like to sit somewhere where it wasn't too crowded. She directed me to a mauve leather chair that reclined and she brought me some ice chips. She offered me other snacks and every beverage under the sun. I declined. I was kind of nervous about what was going to happen. I didn't want to be distracted with a lot of stuff.

My nurse came over to introduce himself—Mack. He verified my name and the type of chemotherapy I will be receiving and then ran off to retrieve the drugs. When he came back he explained to me the process of administering the drugs. He would deliver the three anti-emetics (anti-nausea) first and then FEC.

So as these medicines proceeded to infiltrate my body I had time to observe my surroundings. I was in a place that I would become all too familiar with over the next few months. There were cubicles on all four walls. Each had an occupant in a bed who was receiving some sort of treatment. Understandably, most of the occupants were older since treatment tends to have more of an effect on them.

I got a lot of attention while I was sitting there. It's not expected for me to be in that place; at least, not as an occupant of the chair. The time went by quickly, smoothly. Before I knew it, it was time to go. I didn't feel woozy or nauseous. I felt great as a matter of fact. I could've done cartwheels leaving that place. I was supposed to have someone escort me so they can drive me home and I saw no need. I still had things I needed to do. So I got behind the wheel and proceeded to run some errands.

We drove to campus to check-in with folks. I felt so good I convinced my mother that we can go back to Cincinnati that day so we rushed back to my place and packed up. My mother drove the first leg home and we switched at Kentucky Speedway because I was concerned about her shaky hands.

When I switched with her, I was already not feeling that great but I didn't think things would go downhill so fast. I was surprised we made it home in one piece because by the time we pulled into the driveway, I had enough energy to tell my mother that I needed to lay down. I wouldn't admit to her on the road that I felt like horse crap. I ran in the house, up the stairs, and straight to the toilet. I didn't make it.

12.15.07

The ER

D	ECE	MBE	R 20	07		
S	M	T	W	T	F	S
						1
2	3	4	5	6	7	8
9	10	11	12	13	14	15
16	17	18	19	20	21	22
23	24	25	26	27	28	29
30	31					

Medications: Phenergan, Zofran

Treatments: ER visit, IV placement, Catheter

As I made it to the last step... whoosh. Vomit all over the steps and the bathroom floor. Nausea. Vomiting. This would go on for the next several hours. I had some Phenergan I could take for nausea, but I couldn't keep anything down. In between short catnaps I would be vomiting. My mother tried to feed me, but to no avail. She finally decided that this wasn't normal and called the doctor.

> *Once she started throwing up, it seemed like it never stopped. For hours that was all she did. I knew then that I would not be bringing her home after chemo again. Finally, I decided to call the doctor in Louisville and she told me to take her to the emergency room. We went to Jewish Hospital Kenwood. When we reached the desk all I said was, "Today was her first chemo treatment," and they took her right back. This was the first time that I saw my daughter, my baby, as a cancer patient.*

My mother explained what the situation was and the doctor told her to get me to the emergency room immediately. The doctor feared I was dehydrated. My mother doesn't drive well in the dark so she called my aunt and asked if she would take us. Five minutes later my aunt and grandmother were at the front door I was being loaded in the car, still throwing up.

We went to Jewish Hospital Kenwood. There was only one family in the waiting room. My mother damn near carried me to the desk and they asked if I needed a wheelchair. Normally I would've said no, but I knew I wasn't going to make it down the hall. They immediately brought the chair around and wheeled me to the first available bed. My mother stayed behind to take care of paperwork.

They gave me an IV to replenish my fluids. Then some Zofran. When that didn't work they gave me some more Zofran. That really made me sick and thus I began throwing up again. Nothing they gave me would help. Then they gave me Phenergan which normally works for me I just couldn't hold it down in pill form. That seemed to quiet me down. I was drifting in and out of sleep at that point.

Before they would release me they wanted to make sure there was nothing going on with my bladder or liver. Earlier, they asked if I could use the bathroom and I was so sedated that my answer was no because I didn't want to get up. Now they were talking about using a catheter. Not happening, so I damn near jumped out of the bed.

The nurse helped me to the bathroom. She opened the door, guided me in and shut the door behind me. I remember thinking that the door was unlocked and I hoped no one was going to come in. Just then I tripped over one of those large weight scales and damn near busted my head on the sink. Funny, ya think? Not when you are on drugs.

12.27.07

Women's Day

S	M	T	W	T	F	S
					1	
2	3	4	5	6	7	8
9	10	11	12	13	14	15
16	17	18	19	20	21	22
23	24	25	26	27	28	29
30	31					

December 2007

Medications: Neulasta

Treatments: None

I had an appointment back in Louisville. My mother was planning on driving down and spending the night with me. We would then drive back the next day since there would be family in town.

Somehow this quick excursion blossomed into Women's Day. All of the women in my family (me, grandmother, mom, 2 aunts, 2 cousins) were going to spend the night in my one bedroom apartment. This was going to be fun since it would be a family first.

It's hard to get all of us in one place so we would be able to bond, if only for one night. We had planned on going to the doctor and then going shopping for a few hours and then hitting the road. That plan was foiled when we found out we had to take my god children. These are some busy kids. They require a lot of attention.

I found out that my white blood count was very, very low. The doctor was surprised that I had not gotten sick or had a fever. He told me that the next go round that I would have to get a Neulasta shot. This shot would help boost my immune system. Things did not go as planned, but it was an interesting time. After the doctor, someone decided that we should go to Cracker Barrel. We spent almost two hours there. That left only forty-five minutes for shopping. We headed back to my house to pick up our belongings and hit the road.

1.02.08

Acupuncture

S	M	T	W	T	F	S
		1	2	3	4	5
6	7	8	9	10	11	12
13	14	15	16	17	18	19
20	21	22	23	24	25	26
27	28	29	30	31		

January 2008

Medications: None

Treatments: Acupuncture

The last chemo left me vomiting and nauseous. I was determined that would not happen this time. I was going to do anything in my power to make sure it wasn't going to happen again.

Over the Christmas break, I looked up some acupuncturists in Louisville. My mother had tried this in the past for her colitis and I thought it would be worth a try for nausea. The woman I found was located in a Yoga place down the street from my house. She was shorter than I thought, but I hoped she knew what she was doing.

She led me to a private room and had me sit down on a bed. She gathered detailed information about my history. She explained the process of acupuncture to me and then we talked about different ways I could help myself to assist the acupuncture process. She talked about different herbal treatments I could use for symptoms I was suffering.

She turned on the soothing music and lit some incense. She had me lay down on the bed and began to place the needles. She put one in my abdomen, chest, left wrist, one in each shin, one in each foot and two in my right wrist. She left those in for a few minutes and then came back to stimulate them. She did this by twisting them a little further into my skin. When she twisted the ones in my feet it sent an electrical shockwave through my entire foot. That was one of the weirdest feelings I had ever experienced. She also taped 4 seeds in each ear. When I feel nauseous, I am supposed to rub these.

It was unorthodox, but I was willing to try it. We'll see what tomorrow brings.

1.03.08

Chemo Day 2

S	M	T	W	T	F	S
		1	2	3	4	5
6	7	8	9	10	11	12
13	14	15	16	17	18	19
20	21	22	23	24	25	26
27	28	29	30	31		

JANUARY 2008

Medications: FEC, Aloxi, Emend

Treatments: Chemotherapy

This day started out uneventfully. My mother and aunt came down to Louisville with me for support. I had my blood taken and had to see the doctor as usual. Since the last chemo sent me to the ER, the doctor prescribed an anti-nausea med called Emend.

It was 3 pills. The first I would take an hour before receiving chemo. The next I would take over the course of the next two days. Just a few minutes after the Aloxi (another anti-nausea med) I had the most intense stomach cramps. They were so intense that they had to move me to a bed. Of course, that didn't stop the cramps. I felt like I had to use the bathroom so I did the only thing I could...I crapped (on the toilet). That made me feel better, but the damage was done.

The nurse went to consult the doctor. They asked if I wanted to come back tomorrow. I told the nurse I was going to 'man up' and finish this today. I was not going through that twice. They began giving me saline. Shortly after, they finished pushing through the rest of the meds. I was weak.

I don't remember next 36 hours. I slept much and ate little. Did the acupuncture work? Who knows?

1.08.08

Argh!!

	JANUARY 2008					
S	M	T	W	T	F	S
		1	2	3	4	5
6	7	8	9	10	11	12
13	14	15	16	17	18	19
20	21	22	23	24	25	26
27	28	29	30	31		

Medications: Neupogen

Treatments: None

This word alone should tell you the tone of this particular entry. I am so sick and tired of this crap. How I long for the day when I don't have to remember I have breast cancer. This day has been particularly challenging because I spent all night tossing and turning from hot flashes. I can't sleep hot, so I toss and turn. Then I immediately get the chills. This cycles all day long and prevents me from getting proper rest. It just makes everything that much worse.

Today I had to go back to CBC for a shot of Neupogen. This drug is supposed to help my body produce white blood cells faster. I have to get one every day this week. As I was sitting in the waiting room for my shot, I became anxious. I cannot express properly in words how I feel about needles and IVs. The anticipation drives me nuts. Regardless, I am allowed to feel some moments of melancholy. My emotional and physical state was detectable by more than just my mother because two nurses inquired as to what was wrong. All I could say was that I didn't feel well. After receiving today's shot in the arm, I began to feel hot and I couldn't breathe. It wasn't the medicine in the shot, it was my mind. I was making this much worse but it began to manifest itself physically. I couldn't breathe on the elevator. I practically ran out of the elevator to get fresh air. I had to sit down on the bench and wait for my mother to get the car.

When I got in the car my mother was on the cell with my stepfather. I picked up the phone and began talking to him because she was trying to turn the corner. I was telling him how I felt about needles and he began giving me a pep talk. It brought me to tears. These days it does not take much. I had to give the phone back to my mother.

Nothing tastes like it's supposed to. I don't have a metallic taste, but it's a nothing taste. There's absolutely no enjoyment to eating food. My hair is shedding. Luckily, I still have my eyebrows. I'll have to keep praying on that one because I surely can't draw them back in. Two down, four to go. I just don't know how I'm gonna get through it.

Despair. It's hard to look at the glass as 33% full. I reflect on my choice of being in this damn clinical trial and agreeing to treatments. I could've just as easily opted for the American version of this crap and only had 4 treatments. I would've been halfway through by now. Argh.

1.09.08

The Bald And The Beautiful

S	M	T	W	T	F	S
		1	2	3	4	5
6	7	8	9	10	11	12
13	14	15	16	17	18	19
20	21	22	23	24	25	26
27	28	29	30	31		

JANUARY 2008

Medications: None

Treatments: Haircut

Yup, today I did it.

It is all gone.

After this last chemo treatment, my hair began to shed more and more every day. I could feel an ache in my scalp which signaled to me that the hair was just leaping off my head. By this morning, most of the hair immediately north of my forehead was gone. It was time to do the inevitable.

My stepfather was coming down to Louisville to get my mom (because it was time for her to go). We had him bring the clippers with him. I was worried that it would be traumatic for them seeing the rest of my hair go bye-bye.

As he began to shave off my texturized hair, I felt nothing. What was there to feel? I really thought when the time came that I would be grieving a loss, but seriously I'm cool. I will admit it is a different look for me. Hell, I would go outside like this 1) if it wasn't cold as hell and 2) if it wouldn't bring about attention. I like to be low-key so I'll be sporting the wigs daily now.

I felt liberated before...now I feel even more free. After all I've been through these past few months, a bald head ain't setting me back.

1.22.08

The Birthday Girl

S	M	T	W	T	F	S
		1	2	3	4	5
6	7	8	9	10	11	12
13	14	15	16	17	18	19
20	21	22	23	24	25	26
27	28	29	30	31		

JANUARY 2008

Medications: None

Treatments: None

Well, I made it to 32. I'm so glad to not be 31 anymore. Kisha was diagnosed with Lupus at 31. Ebony had some serious issues that put her in the hospital at 31. There's something about prime numbers that spell disaster. But I digress and won't go into my personal theories.

People asked what I did for my birthday. I actually have never celebrated my birthday on my birthday because it usually doesn't fall on a weekend. I celebrate with Dr. King since everyone is off that day. I prepared for chemo. I drove from Cincy to Louisville with my mom. We did our usual pre-chemo errands (grocery store, etc.) and settled down for the evening. Some birthday, huh?

1.29.08

Chemo 3 & The Sinus Infection

S	M	T	W	T	F	S
		1	2	3	4	5
6	7	8	9	10	11	12
13	14	15	16	17	18	19
20	21	22	23	24	25	26
27	28	29	30	31		

JANUARY 2008

Medications: FEC, Neupogen, Mucinex, Tussionex, Theraflu, Avelox

Treatments: Chemotherapy

I was kind of uneasy going into this treatment. If you remember last time, I tried acupuncture to help ease the nausea. I'm not sure if it worked or not but I decided not to have it this time. I'm kinda playing trial and error with some things to see what works best. The one thing I knew for sure was that they wouldn't be putting any more Aloxi in my body. Those stomach cramps were out of control.

My anxiety was also getting out of hand. I didn't really know what to expect with the last two treatments, but by now this thing should be old hat. Getting my mind under control would be my goal to also help control the nausea. Just even walking into the CBC would make me sick. Mind over matter, right?

Surprisingly enough, this chemo went fairly well. I don't remember much from it so that's good! I spent most of the time asleep in the chair because they gave me the good stuff. No nausea, no vomiting, no stomach cramps. I came home and slept it off. I couldn't ask for a better time.

I still have to go for my Neupogen shots everyday this week to help increase my white blood cells. I've gotten quite used to the needle sticks every day in the back of my arm. For the last 10 days I've been sick. I've been treating what I thought was a cold. I think it began that way and then it morphed into a sinus infection. I have spent the last 10 days without sleep, coughing my head off, and mucus coming out of my damn eyes. I had been taking TheraFlu daytime and nighttime. Usually the nighttime stuff makes me go to sleep, but that stuff didn't even phase me. I began taking Mucinex for the mucus, but it was still out of hand. We called the doctor over the weekend and he prescribed Tussionex to help with the coughs. He told me that it has a narcotic in it and I may not want to drive due to drowsiness. Everyday that I went in to get my Neupogen shots, the nurse would look at me and she could tell that things weren't going well.

Finally, after some consultation with the nurse practitioner they figured out that I developed a sinus infection. Yay, my first one! They prescribed me some Avelox and things are clearing up. I'm hoping to get back to my semi-normal activities beginning next week and we'll see what happens. Once I get rid of this sinus infection, I'll be 100% better.

2.01.08

Chemotherapy's Midpoint Evaluation

FEBRUARY 2008						
S	M	T	W	T	F	S
					1	2
3	4	5	6	7	8	9
10	11	12	13	14	15	16
17	18	19	20	21	22	23
24	25	26	27	28	29	

Medications: None

Treatments: None

"Hi. Chemo here! I've been ravaging your body 7 weeks now. Your body has been overloaded with a myriad number of destructive drugs to kill every last healthy cell in your body. I want to check my work. Let's run through the checklist:

- Hair loss - massive evacuation of all follicles resulting in hair leaping from the body as if on fire

* Bonus (+2): complete eradication of all hair including arm and knuckle hair

- Tastebuds - inability to appreciate anything with flavor

- White blood count - plummet to the depths of hell in order to make subject susceptible to every germ known to man

- Diarrhea/Constipation - spending absurd amounts of time visiting the porcelain god while in a sitting position

*Bonus (+1): grunting involved

- Fatigue - turn subject into a recluse by making sure she can't reach people in the outside world

- Menopausal symptoms - bring on hot flashes close to the point of spontaneous combustion

- Infertility - make sure the subject is unable to continue the bloodline by pillaging every egg in the village (ok, ovaries)

- Penalty (-2): some eggs escape by hiding

- Dry mouth - make it difficult for the subject to communicate with others by eliminating all saliva from the mouth

*Bonus (+1): mouth sores

- Nausea/vomiting - spending absurd amounts of time visiting the porcelain god while sitting on the floor in a leaning position

- Penalty (~2): subject-induced

- Weight gain - add insult to injury by making sure the subject has to buy a new wardrobe because she can't fit her clothes anymore.

- Penalty (-1): weight loss

- Pain - mild to severe bouts of pain in random parts of the body at random intervals, sort of like the old Simon Says game

*Bonus (+1): causing pain to the flap of skin between the big toe and the first toe

Note to Mr. B. Cancer, supervisor: This subject has proven to be difficult. Though this is only the mid-point evaluation, it doesn't look like we're making much progress. We may have to call this one a loss. I will keep trying, but I am not hopeful as to a positive end result from a cancer/chemo point of view."

2.01.08

30th Installment!

S	M	T	W	T	F	S
					1	2
3	4	5	6	7	8	9
10	11	12	13	14	15	16
17	18	19	20	21	22	23
24	25	26	27	28	29	

February 2008

Medications: None

Treatments: None

It's only right that my 30th blog post be filled with some comedy! I had the biggest laugh today that I've had in a very long time. Luckily, I still have a good sense of humor.

Today, I went condo shopping with my aunt. My mother, grandmother, and other aunt were also present. We pulled into the visitor's parking and got out of the car. Where we parked was next to a steep hill that was heavily wooded.

Just as I got out of the car a strong gust of wind blew and ripped the wig off of my head. I shouted to my grandmother, who was still getting out of the car, to get that. She didn't know I meant my hair so she didn't react fast enough. I knew that if the wind kept blowing that my wig was going to be in the woods. My silly self throws my body on the ground to keep the wig from going over the hill.

My mother realized what was going on and began blocking me from view. I still had my stocking cap on, but I couldn't manage to get the wig back on because I was laughing too hard. I finally made it back in the car where I had to wipe away my tears of laughter before I could put it back on.

My aunt gave me a bobby pin, but now that I think about it there's nothing to even bobby pin the wig too. I don't have any hair!!! If ya'll could've been there, you would've been on the ground cracking up. Just hilarious!

2.19.08

Chemo 4

FEBRUARY 2008						
S	M	T	W	T	F	S
					1	2
3	4	5	6	7	8	9
10	11	12	13	14	15	16
17	18	19	20	21	22	23
24	25	26	27	28	29	

Medications: FEC, Neupogen

Treatments: Chemotherapy

The fourth chemo was par for the course. It wasn't the best chemo, but it wasn't the worst. It's taking me a bit longer to recover because me and my mom both forgot that I had some medicine I needed to take to prevent nausea. How can you forget one asks? That's relatively easy since I chose to be asleep for about 36 hours afterward. I don't remember to do anything, including use the bathroom or eat for a day and a half following chemo.

I still have to get my Neupogen shots following chemo. Over the weekend I had to go to the hospital to get them since the CBC is closed. When I went on Saturday everybody and their mother was there, literally. I was there over an hour because somehow I didn't get lab work done at CBC the previous day and I had to wait.

They put everyone in the same room in the Oncology department. I hate hospitals. It's hard enough visiting the CBC every day, but to have to sit in a room with people receiving blood transfusions kind of made my stomach turn. Yes, I'm squeamish if you hadn't figured that out.

Contrary to popular belief (I've always wanted to use that phrase), overexposure to something does not always help you adjust to something. I don't want this experience to be normalized.

I'll be getting back to campus on Wednesday. I still have to take it easy though. One day at a time.

2.19.08

Body Image

| FEBRUARY 2008 |||||||
S	M	T	W	T	F	S
					1	2
3	4	5	6	7	8	9
10	11	12	13	14	15	16
17	18	19	20	21	22	23
24	25	26	27	28	29	

Medications: None

Treatments: None

Many of you have invested hours reading these damn blogs and it would be unfair to censor my thoughts. Some things are just personal and step outside the boundary of what others need to know. Ahh, here goes...

I was in the bathroom the other day and happened to look at my naked self in the mirror.

I noticed that my left nipple is now larger than my right nipple. The left breast is the one that's been poked and prodded the most from the biopsies and lumpectomy. No one told me that this particular kind of oddity would result. I don't like it. I'm not happy with it at all.

I'm fairly certain that my breast size has not changed although I can feel where scar tissue has developed within the breast. It's a lot firmer than it used to be.

Along with everything else that's happening to my body, I now have to figure out how to deal with a big ass nipple. My nipples were fine in proportion to the size of my breast. It's like having an alien sitting there on my breast. Okay, I might be over-descriptive, but I'm trying to drive home a point. I'm annoyed. Every woman has their issues with body image, but I almost wished I hadn't looked in the mirror that day. Argh...

2.20.08

It's Mastectomy & Reconstruction

	FEBRUARY 2008					
S	M	T	W	T	F	S
					1	2
3	4	5	6	7	8	9
10	11	12	13	14	15	16
17	18	19	20	21	22	23
24	25	26	27	28	29	

Medications: None

Treatments: Mastectomy, Reconstruction, Radiation

I'm about 95% sure that this summer I will be having a bilateral mastectomy and reconstruction. This is something I've been considering since doing my research into how to be proactive in preventing a reoccurrence. No method is 100% foolproof, but I'm going to do what I have to do not to go through this again.

After talking to my oncologist, I've got two choices. I can either do 5 or 6 weeks of radiation therapy immediately following chemo and then wait 3 to 6 months to do the mastectomy/reconstruction, OR I can forego radiation therapy and have the mastectomy/reconstruction soon after chemo.

I would have to schedule the surgery for after I take comps (exams) because I cannot postpone this crap any longer. I won't go into the gruesome details now, but I will after I meet with my surgical oncologist and my plastic surgeon.

3.04.08

Why Thinking Before You Speak Is A Good Idea

MARCH 2008

S	M	T	W	T	F	S
						1
2	3	4	5	6	7	8
9	10	11	12	13	14	15
16	17	18	19	20	21	22
23	24	25	26	27	28	29
30	31					

Medications: None

Treatments: None

I know people mean well, but I've had people say some very random and slightly inappropriate things to me since I've been diagnosed.

Others: "My (Insert relative here) had cancer, but s/he died."

Okay, let's think about this for a minute....

Time's up! I don't need to hear about any relatives who have died of cancer. Seriously, is that meant to be a pick me up? More appropriate might be a success story. I want to know about people who are alive and kicking. People just don't think.

Me: "I found a lump"

Others: "Oh, you'll be alright. I had a lump a few years ago and it was just fluke."

I cannot tell you how many folks shared their lump stories with me. What I repeated most often to people was that *my* lump is not *their* lump. Just because it was fine for them, doesn't mean it would be fine for me.

Others: "If you need anything, give me a call."

Sounds good, doesn't it? I've had everyone and their dog say this to me. I don't complain and I don't ask for much help because that's not who I am, but if you want to give me something... **give it!** Don't make me ask for it. Ya'll know I'm in need. I am a full-time student whose expenses outweigh my income. I need money. I accept any American currency, Kroger gift certificates, Walgreens Gift certificates, etc. I like to eat so I accept food also. For those of you who have donated to the EJH Fund, I appreciate it.

It drives me crazy that even now, 5 months after my diagnosis, that the only topic some people talk to me about is cancer. Really, I recognize that I am the afflicted, but do you think I want to talk about this every day at every possible moment?? I cherish the times (albeit they are few) when I can forget that I'm in the midst of battle. I need diversions more than anything else, not reminders. I'm looking for normalcy.

Others: "How are you doing?"
Me: "I'm good"
Others: "No really, how are you doing?"

Must I be broken down and a recluse lying on my floor crying all the time? Having cancer sucks! Enduring chemotherapy and its side effects suck! At any given point in time, something is probably wrong, but I'll be damned if I'm gonna complain about it. I have all my limbs and other than having cancer, I'm perfectly healthy. Even worse than that, usually when people ask how you are doing they are not prepared to hear the actual answer.

Worse than saying something boneheaded is not saying anything at all. To be honest, this is hurtful. I've had people I've been friends with for years and they haven't communicated with me at all since my diagnosis. I can empathize with not knowing what to say to someone who may have received bad news or is mourning, but...to say nothing at all? You can go online and find good things and not-so-good things to say to someone. You can ask people who've endured something, "what's good to say?"

Others: "It'll grow back."

This, of course, is a reference to the hair on my head. I know that it will grow back, but it doesn't help me deal with the loss. Is this revelation supposed to make me feel better? Do you know how long it'll take to get my hair back to the length it once was? Wearing a wig is not really a great solution because anyone who's worn them knows that those things are hot!! I can't wait to come home and pull that wig off every day!

MY BURDENS

My burdens are sometimes heavy
And I often feel alone
Because when I need a friend to lift me up
Nobody's home

I suffer from independence
Which is usually a positive trait
No one worries about me
I'm the one who won't break

Truth is...I have my breaking points
And sometimes I need an ear
Just want someone to talk to
About my hopes and my fears

When life seems too much to bear
Within myself I retreat
There I seek peace
That is where I will be replete

When I emerge from my shell
People rush to ask what's wrong
But if you had been there before I went in
You would've known all along

My burdens are sometimes heavy
I'll be fine because I know
God wouldn't put anything on me
That I couldn't handle

3.10.08

Chemo 5

	MARCH 2008					
S	M	T	W	T	F	S
						1
2	3	4	5	6	7	8
9	10	11	12	13	14	15
16	17	18	19	20	21	22
23	24	25	26	27	28	29
30	31					

Medications: Neulasta, Neupogen

Treatments: None

Well, this one went as normal as possible. It was the aftermath that was not normal. Per usual, the first two days I slept. On day three, I was moving around a little, but felt nauseous. I was taking my prescribed medicine, but it didn't help very much. By the time I got to day four, it was unbearable and I slept all that day too. On day five the nausea was bearable and finally went away on day six.

This time instead of getting the series of shots (Neupogen) to increase my white blood cell count, I had them give me Neulasta. Neulasta is good because I only have to get one shot, but it causes bone pain. I was having bone pain with the Neupogen also, so I figured why not go for it. Last time I had to get a series of 10 shots which means I had to visit the CBC each day for 10 days. That's excluding the weekend because they're not open so I would have to go the hospital. The thing about going to the hospital is that they charge more than the CBC just to give me one shot. The difference in the charges is ridiculous. Seriously.

3.14.08

More Decisions

	MARCH 2008					
S	M	T	W	T	F	S
						1
2	3	4	5	6	7	8
9	10	11	12	13	14	15
16	17	18	19	20	21	22
23	24	25	26	27	28	29
30	31					

Medications: None

Treatments: Mastectomy, Reconstruction, Chemo, Genetic Testing

I've had a series of meetings with my surgical oncologist, plastic surgeon, and my oncologist. I will be having my bilateral mastectomy and reconstruction on July 2nd. I'm excited. It's allowing me to look beyond this last chemo.

Everything seems to be falling into place. My work fellowship requires me to be full-time so I have to take a class this summer. Fortunately, the class is in the beginning part of the summer and won't interfere with anything. Having the surgery at the beginning of July is ideal because I should be back up and running when classes begin in the fall. The stars have aligned.

I've also decided to have genetic testing. I'm not having it for me though. Since I am the only one who's been fortunate enough (sarcasm) to be diagnosed with any kind of cancer in my family, I I feel like I need to figure out if I inherited some mutant gene or if I'm the mutant. My biggest concern with genetic testing was discrimination. I had heard lots of different things from different people regarding disclosure to employers. If I was found to have the gene, I didn't know how that would affect my job search. I finally just called a genetic counselor at the hospital and had a phone consultation. She answered all of my questions and that led to my decision to move forward with the tests. Those damn tests are expensive. We're talking over $3,000. Luckily, my insurance company will pay 90%. Normally, someone would have the testing done prior to being diagnosed especially if other members of their family had cancer. My surgeon recommended I get testing to help me decide whether I should get a bilateral mastectomy. I'm not trying to have cancer again so I am pulling out all the stops.

So, the results of the genetic testing won't affect any of my future decisions because I intend to be as proactive as possible. I've already decided to have my ovaries removed at some point down the road - ovarian cancer is a monster. I still hold out hope for now that my ovaries will regain their function once chemo has been completed.

Even though no one else in my family has been diagnosed, it doesn't mean that the gene wasn't passed along. The genetic testing won't be specific enough to tell me which side of the family it came from, if at all. Nevertheless, if the gene was inherited it will put the rest of my family on notice. It will motivate them to have better screenings. It will allow me to know if I might pass the gene onto my children (if I have any).

My mother mentioned that she might not want to know the results, but from my point of view, I don't want to watch anybody else in my family go through what I've been through. Knowledge is power. I'm gonna have to steal a line from GI Joe....'Knowing is half the battle.'

4.14.08

The Finale

April 2008						
S	M	T	W	T	F	S
		1	2	3	4	5
6	7	8	9	10	11	12
13	14	15	16	17	18	19
20	21	22	23	24	25	26
27	28	29	30			

Medications: FEC, Emend, Neulasta, Neupogen

Treatments: Mastectomy, Reconstruction

So, it's been a good minute since my last blog entry. To tell you the truth, this last chemo was a doozy! I found out a couple of days before my last chemo that I had met my prescription limit. That's unfortunate considering it's only April. There's a drug, Emend, that I take to help with the nausea. I take it over a course of 3 days beginning one hour prior to chemo. Well, this drug normally costs about $400. Who doesn't have $400 is me.

In the meantime, I had gone to a conference in Atlanta. My mom did the leg work to try to get the doctor's office to provide me with some samples of something in place of the Emend. After hours of begging, she was able to get them to give me samples. They didn't work. I did more vomiting on this chemo than any other time except of the first time. I was sick as a dog for about six days. I slept the first two days, the fourth day, and half of the fifth day to avoid the nausea. Then, I was extremely fatigued for a few days after that. I sent my mom packing on day four because it was easier to have someone come and get her on a Sunday.

Since this was my last chemo I wasn't required to get Neupogen or Neulasta shots. My white blood count (WBC) would remain low and bounce back on its own. Unfortunately, my WBC tanks out to almost nothing. I am now going to the CBC on a weekly basis for lab work.

I am now preparing for the next step in this grueling saga ... Bilateral mastectomy & reconstruction. Be there or be square July 2, 2008...

4.18.08

12 Reasons Why I Love Chemo!

	APRIL 2008					
S	M	T	W	T	F	S
		1	2	3	4	5
6	7	8	9	10	11	12
13	14	15	16	17	18	19
20	21	22	23	24	25	26
27	28	29	30			

Medications: None

Treatments: None

Ok, who really loves chemo? Nobody, but I was forced to find a silver lining on this smoky gray cloud.

1. I love chemo for taking my hair. I'm hoping that the new growth will display my rumored 'Asian roots' and I won't have to relax my hair ever again. Thanks Chemo!
2. I love chemo for taking the 'right' hair. I prayed about not losing my eyebrows and the Lord granted that wish. My hair is starting to grow back now and my armpit hair hasn't grown back in. I'm hoping it doesn't come back. Thanks Chemo!
3. I love chemo for taking away my migraines. I haven't had a migraine since this nightmare began. How marvelous! For any migraine sufferer, you know that's major. Thanks Chemo!
4. I love chemo for letting me be lazy. Okay, so I was already lazy, but what better excuse to lie around all day. People have been at my beck and call for the last few months. I almost felt like royalty. Thanks Chemo!

5. I love chemo for making me drink water. Seriously, my water intake was close to nil. My body needed the water. It's healthier. Thanks Chemo!
6. I love chemo for bringing me back to an exercise regimen. Because my energy level was low and my hormones are out of whack, the need to exercise increased. Even though I am not doing very much exercising, I have begun walking again. Thanks Chemo!
7. I love chemo for allowing me time to write. Because I am so busy I haven't had time to write. Blogging has allowed me to open up emotionally to myself and others. That's major considering I'm a thinker and not a feeler. Thanks Chemo!
8. I love chemo for allowing me to get closer to some family members. It sucks that it takes something like this for that to happen, but sometimes the reason doesn't matter. Thanks Chemo!
9. I love chemo for helping me get a handicap tag so I can park closer to the buildings I need to do business in! Thanks Chemo!

10. I love chemo for allowing me to experience what it's like to take a shower without a shower cap. The water feels awesome pouring down over my head and onto my shoulders. Thanks Chemo!
11. I love chemo for making me eat healthier. During chemo I didn't drink pop and cut out certain foods that were blowing up my cholesterol. Overall, my diet is now just a tad bit healthier. Thanks Chemo!
12. I love chemo for allowing me to redirect my energies. I've reprioritized some things in my life. I have a better grip on what I need to do. It's given me reason to shed unnecessary baggage. Thanks Chemo!

4.20.08

Finding The Joy In Trying Times

APRIL 2008

S	M	T	W	T	F	S
		1	2	3	4	5
6	7	8	9	10	11	12
13	14	15	16	17	18	19
20	21	22	23	24	25	26
27	28	29	30			

Medications: None

Treatments: None

Considering that this has been the worst experience of my life, I was able to remain positive and whoop this cancer's ass! I am by no means an optimist, but I view many things now through a different lens.

I have experienced the generosity of others. My mother has spent countless hours taking care of me. She relocated to Louisville for a week every 3 weeks for me. She fed me, held me, made sure I took my meds, and sat patiently by my side while I received chemo (and countless other things). For that I am incredibly thankful.

I have had many strangers donate money to my cause or just keep me in their prayers. My mother's former supervisor sent me a card damn near every week letting me know that she was thinking about me. I am so amazed that people who don't even know me would want to contribute to my plight. There have been fundraisers done at the Post Office and a raffle my family coordinated. To those of you who have spoken kind words to me or just checked to see how I'm doing, I thank you. To those folks who have not reached out to me during this time or were slow in communicating with me, it's okay really. Sometimes it's hard to find the words to say. Hearing about someone else's issues can often bring on thoughts of your own mortality. I understand. It doesn't make me think you care any less. It's all good! I appreciate more things and at the same time I don't sweat the petty stuff. Life is too short to be dealing with silly crap. It's time for the excess baggage to go. I'm working on improving my relationships with those I truly care about. I not only view life differently, I view myself differently. I've been able to observe myself through the eyes of others. My faith and inner strength have really emerged during this time. I believe my life philosophy and my personality have helped me to maintain my sanity.

I will admit that I checked out (mentally) from October through March. While still in pursuit of my education, I didn't care as much. Sometimes I made it to campus, sometimes I didn't. My perspective about what's important changed. Concentrating on anything was a no go. It took me quite a while to regain my focus, but I have it back now. Even though I won't be graduating in the time originally planned, I will finish. Everything in its time.

See you after surgery. To be continued......

5.07.08

What I Wanna Say...

May 2008

S	M	T	W	T	F	S
				1	2	3
4	5	6	7	8	9	10
11	12	13	14	15	16	17
18	19	20	21	22	23	24
25	26	27	28	29	30	31

Medications: None

Treatments: Intimacy Issues

Being intimate with someone has been furthest from my mind since this whole ordeal began. Besides, I didn't even think anyone would wanna be involved with me or that I could still be attractive to someone while like this: no hair, scars all over, a few pounds heavier than normal.

When I was propositioned, I found myself saying to this person that I wasn't ready. I said I wasn't ready because I wanted to grow hair first. I didn't mean to say it out loud, but it was the truth. I feel so far from being a sexual being. This person was being sensitive to my needs. He asked what I needed from him and if it would make me feel more comfortable I could wear a scarf. It's a lot to ask of someone. It's one thing to reveal yourself by being intimate with someone, it's another to show yourself this way. I don't really carry many self-esteem issues, but I am now finding that I may have intimacy problems right now. I don't know how my body will react. Will I be able to go for a long time? Will I be able to naturally moisten? It's a lot to think about

I'm still back to trust. Am I willing to extend this kind of trust to him? Do I even want to do this myself. Casual sex...not the most appealing idea. I don't want my heart broken to fulfill a temporary need that I don't currently have at the moment. Would he be willing to settle for less? It seems a conversation is necessary...

7.01.08

Mastectomy & Reconstruction

	JULY 2008					
S	M	T	W	T	F	S
		1	2	3	4	5
6	7	8	9	10	11	12
13	14	15	16	17	18	19
20	21	22	23	24	25	26
27	28	29	30	31		

Medications: None

Treatments: Mastectomy and Reconstruction

Tomorrow I go in for my bilateral mastectomy and reconstruction. I am getting a little anxious. I really just want to get it over with. I'm not looking forward to the pain. I really don't know what to expect though. I haven't spoken with anyone at length about the process because since I have to go through it anyway, I don't want to psych myself out.

My entire family will be coming to Louisville to support me. My parents will be coming down shortly and my grandmother and aunts will be here later tonight. Tomorrow Kisha will be making an appearance as well. We'll see how we all hold up with 10 folks in my one bedroom apartment.

I'm not thrilled that the surgery doesn't actually begin until 1pm, meaning that I have to be at the hospital by 11am. I can't eat after midnight the night before so I will be incredibly hungry all morning. I've instructed my mother not to wake me up before 10:30am because I don't want to have time to get hungry.

7.02.08

It's Surgery Day!!!

	JULY 2008					
S	M	T	W	T	F	S
	1	2	3	4	5	
6	7	8	9	10	11	12
13	14	15	16	17	18	19
20	21	22	23	24	25	26
27	28	29	30	31		

Medications: Anesthesia

Treatments: Bilateral Mastectomies, IV Placement

It's surgery day! Mostly everyone was there with the exception of the Jordans. I got up at the last minute because I didn't want to be too hungry. I left post-it notes for myself on the doors reminding myself not to eat and not to use the bathroom. I was instructed that I would have to give a urine sample upon arrival and since I had not drank anything I only had one shot.

It was a bit of a mad house in the living room. They were all running around and attempting to be quiet while I slept. We caravanned to the hospital. I rode with Kisha to the hospital. When we arrived the other two cars were able to find a parking place, but we couldn't find one. I jumped out in the parking garage so I wouldn't be late, and had Nina and ReRe go with her to find a parking place while I checked in.

I checked in as soon as I arrived. I carried with me my pink Tweety Bird socks. I requested a private room and then asked if I could give my urine sample right then because I had to use the bathroom really bad. Upon my return to the desk, the nurse was already ready for me to check in. I gave my mother a hug and kiss and the nurse took me in the back. I was led to the equivalent of a hospital cubicle. It was the size of a jail cell with one wall being curtained. The nurse began to ask me questions I had already answered the previous week at my pre-op appointment. She confirmed with me that I knew which procedure I was there for and who my surgeons were. During the conversation I had to be firm with the nurse. Even though I was having a mastectomy done on both sides, that didn't mean it was equal opportunity to use either arm during surgery. Since I had a lumpectomy on the left side in October means that I will never be able to have a blood pressure cuff or a needle stick in that arm. I had to make sure that she marked my left arm so that nurses and doctors would know not to venture there.

The worst part of all this for me is the insertion of the IV. I hated needles before and my disgust hasn't improved. The veins in my right arm still aren't completely healed. When I look down at my arm, I see burned and dry veins. Being light-complexioned doesn't help either. Evidence of chemo is apparent. Drawing blood or inserting an IV into the tired veins in my right arm is a task, but it has to be that arm. It has to be closer to the hand to be effective. The thing that kills me is that in order to insert the IV into the hand they have to shoot you with a numbing agent first. Once the IV was in, I basically sat back and waited for time to go by. They allow your family members to come back in pairs at that point. My family never follows instructions. They disobey the two-person-only rule. My mother and grandmother were the first to come back. Then Kisha wandered back there. She led us in a prayer that made me shed a tear. Even though Kisha had made me mad the week before, the love I have for her overshadowed that and melted away the anger. The rest of my family came back. They always try to make me laugh. I had less fear this time around. I'm always worried about not waking up, but if I didn't I wouldn't know it anyway. After family time, the nurse came to wheel me out. I said my I love you and goodbyes. I can never figure out how they seem to remember how to get where. They wheel you down and around corridors, get on an elevator, and go down some more corridors.

We arrived at the surgery room. It was cold and sterile. I didn't see either of my surgeons. I remember them pushing the anesthesia in and then it was lights out. The surgery took about 5 hours. My general surgeon went in and performed the mastectomies and my plastic surgeon put everything back together after inserting the tissue expanders. Kisha came in while I was still in recovery to say goodbye. It was going to be getting dark soon and she had to work the next day. She drove back to Cincy. When I finally woke up, I was in my private room, number 665. I slept mostly. When I wasn't sleeping I was throwing up. My body doesn't like anesthesia so it gets rid of it, I think I threw up about five times. I would point to my mouth and my mother instantly knew what was going to happen.

As the night progressed, it seemed as if a nurse came in the room every hour to check my vitals. As a result, sleep was not restful. My mother ended up staying with me all night. She slept in a chair. I know that must've been uncomfortable. At 6:00 am she told me that she was leaving and would be back in a little while. She wanted to go wash up and change clothes. She's a light sleeper, so I'm fairly certain she didn't get much sleep either.

At about 7:30 am or 8:00 am food service came in with breakfast. She just dropped it off. I tried to maneuver myself so I could eat but was having the damnedest time. I didn't really have great use of my arms, shoulders, or chest area in general so I had to improvise. I was very frustrated. I was mad at my mother for not coming back because I needed her help to eat and she was not there.

I managed to eat some of the nasty scrambled eggs. It appeared that the doctors put me on a no-substance diet because I had been throwing up the night before. I could barely get the cranberry juice open because it was in a peel back container. I cannot convey to you the frustration I felt not being able to eat and not being able to use my arms.

My mother and my cousin Gina came to the hospital at 10:00 am. I was happy and mad. I told them of the saga that happened involving my breakfast, which at that point seemed like it had been many hours ago. I had complaints because the nursing staff didn't come when called. I was annoyed.

Two of the administrative assistants from University of Louisville came to visit me at the hospital. They came bearing many gifts. Many of the professors bought me knick knacks to help cheer me up. I was told that I could only open one per day. They didn't stay very long, but it was a bright spot in my day. My advisor also came to the hospital to see me. He had called earlier on my cell phone to let me know that he was coming.

I have never had a stranger bathe me before. While it was a little odd, I almost didn't care. You do what has to be done. She asked if I wanted to wash my own private parts and I said yes. I had enough mobility for that. I knew she was willing to do it, but why have someone else do it when you can do it yourself?

My surgeons did come in at least once to check on me. That was more than I expected considering that is was near the July 4th holiday. I only stayed in the hospital two nights. Insurance makes sure you stay for the least amount of time possible. The next day or so was uneventful. They continued to serve me nasty food and the nurses came in every hour to get my vitals. During that time my family members visited. My two godchildren were at my house and I'm glad they didn't have them come to the hospital. I want them minimally exposed to what I've been going through.

7.04.08

I'm Going Home

JULY 2008

S	M	T	W	T	F	S
		1	2	3	4	5
6	7	8	9	10	11	12
13	14	15	16	17	18	19
20	21	22	23	24	25	26
27	28	29	30	31		

Medications: Pain Medicine

Treatments: None

I was still on some good pain medicine. I didn't feel much pain, but I was uncomfortable. The bumps from the drive were sort of painful. I wouldn't be able to shower for a few days. Bummer.

As soon as I got home, I saw my godchildren, Cameron and Kaylin. They had given the kids instructions not to touch me. Cameron looked like he wanted to hug me and that was okay. I told him he could hug my leg. That was good enough for him.

I went directly to my bedroom to lie down. I didn't really feel like sleeping so I had them set the t.v. set on a chair in the living room. There was no way I was going to get any sleep with all of those people in there. I couldn't do much and everyone wanted to do everything for me. I'm not used to so much attention. I stayed up for quite awhile that day. When nighttime rolled around, I felt bad for hogging the bed all to myself. The next morning I felt stiff. I could only sleep sitting up. So once again, sleep was just as fitful at home as it was in the hospital.

7.15.08

What To Wear?

	JULY 2008					
S	M	T	W	T	F	S
		1	2	3	4	5
6	7	8	9	10	11	12
13	14	15	16	17	18	19
20	21	22	23	24	25	26
27	28	29	30	31		

Medications: None

Treatments: None

I've been struggling trying to find shirts to wear. I can't wear regular t-shirts or tank tops because you can see the straight line from the surgery through my clothes. I haven't been left with a lot of options. I have some sleeveless, button-up shirts that I've been wearing. They are a little loose, but I hate being forced to wear something.

I've gone to the store to find some more tops and I haven't had much luck...everything is spandex. Since I've lived a lazy lifestyle since October, I have gained a few pounds in my mid-section and the spandex tops show everything. Argh!!

7.20.08

Fill Up Time

	JULY 2008					
S	M	T	W	T	F	S
		1	2	3	4	5
6	7	8	9	10	11	12
13	14	15	16	17	18	19
20	21	22	23	24	25	26
27	28	29	30	31		

Medications: None

Treatments: 'Fill-Up'

FILL UP!! I tried to as much as I could to prepare her for her first fill up only to be let down on her first visit because she was still sore and the doctor felt it best not to fill her up today.

The next visit he did fill her up with 50cc's of saline. She could not watch but I watched as he stuck a long needle into her chest. This is what I saw: He took a small oval shaped device that could be held with two fingers, it had a magnet on one side, and placed it on her chest at the top of the implant (tissue expander) and used a marker to place a dot. He did this three times drawing a triangle, which indicates where to stick the needle. He stuck the needle right in the center of the triangle. The needle was long and it was attached to a bag of solution with two tubes - one to suck the solution into the first tube, and the other to release the solution into the needle and the implant. Her chest was still numb from the surgery so she did not even feel the needle going in. All she felt was pressure and she did not look.

It only took ten minutes and it was over. Right after that, she became ill and we had to wait until she calmed down and could walk. She was not supposed to lift more than a gallon of milk. Of course, that meant nothing to her. Life goes on and you forget not to lift.

Now the bandages are off and she's going for her second fill up. She gets 50 more CC's. She did well and now I get to go home. This is the first time in my life that I've been away from home for this long a period of time. I feel like since October I sometimes get to pass through my house, my city or visit my husband. I am slowly picking up my life but sometimes I feel myself just sitting still waiting for her to call. I know I have to go back for another surgery but that's just for the real implants. I'm okay because it's going to be easier for me than for her. All I have to do is sit still and wait. PRAY and wait.

7.25.08

Looking In The Mirror

	JULY 2008					
S	M	T	W	T	F	S
		1	2	3	4	5
6	7	8	9	10	11	12
13	14	15	16	17	18	19
20	21	22	23	24	25	26
27	28	29	30	31		

Medications: None

Treatments: Bandage Removal

I took off my steri-strips today. I've had them on three weeks now and it was about time.

I could see that the scabs wanted to peel off underneath and it was becoming bulky.

I stared at myself in the mirror. Up until now, I didn't have to think about not having nipples because the steri-strips were there. With the steri-strips off, I came face-to-face with what was left. It was strange looking in the mirror. Where there used to be a nipple, there was now a straight line.

No words to describe it perfectly, just odd.

7.26.08

Menses

	JULY 2008					
S	M	T	W	T	F	S
		1	2	3	4	5
6	7	8	9	10	11	12
13	14	15	16	17	18	19
20	21	22	23	24	25	26
27	28	29	30	31		

Medications: None

Treatments: Chemotherapy, Fertility

I began my period today. Not sure how I feel about that. It's been six months since my last one - the chemotherapy put a kibosh on that. I'm feeling pretty crappy right now. It's that 'ugh' feeling that just can't be described any other way. Not only has it come back, it's come back with a vengeance.

The silver lining in this is that reproduction may be on the horizon. I'm quietly excited. I hope that I haven't been rendered sterile as a result of the chemotherapy. I don't want to get my hopes up though. I avoid disappointment by attuning my expectations appropriately. I want to be a mother someday, and maybe God wants me to be a mother, too!

Depression

"…..sometimes when I'm stressed, I pick up a coloring book and some crayons and just color the world away." EJH

3.12.09

My Thoughts

	MARCH 2009					
S	M	T	W	T	F	S
1	2	3	4	5	6	7
8	9	10	11	12	13	14
15	16	17	18	19	20	21
22	23	24	25	26	27	28
29	30	31				

Medications: None

Treatments: None

Things haven't been right with me for a while. I sent an IM to a friend asking for a pep talk. I've known for a long time that I've needed to get my ass in gear, but I was having trouble finding the motivation. I've been doing the very minimum of what has been required of me. My desire to complete this Ph.D. program...does not exist. To be honest, I could take it or leave it. If I finish, great. If I don't finish...oh well.

My desire to produce any jewelry...does not exist. I don't think I could muster any creative juices right now if I tried. My desire to produce any products for 'It's a Pink Thing!'...does not exist. 'How long has this been going on?", you ask. Probably since my diagnosis. I mentally checked out in the middle of my last semester of class work. With the help of my professors, I was able to complete all but one class, in which I currently have an *Incomplete*. He'll get the work when I give it to him.

Since October 2007, life has been moving full speed ahead, going from one surgery/process to the next. Things moved so fast. I didn't have time to spend mourning my diagnosis. I spent my time worried about how I was going to finish this doctoral program, how I was going to pay for these bills, and making sure others were okay.

The friend I IM'ed asked me 'What's wrong?' As I tried to explain to him what was wrong, I came upon the revelation that I was suffering some form of depression. To discover that I might be depressed was a revelation for me. I thought I was dealing with breast cancer well, but I guess I haven't been. I don't quite know when it started, but there's been a progression into absence of productivity. To the average person, it probably looks like I'm functioning fine. To myself and maybe my mother, we knew that something was off.

The last time I felt this way was in college. My roommate's father died. No one close to me has ever died, so I didn't know what she was going through...but his death unexpectedly affected me. She had now lost both of her parents and there was nothing I could do to console her. That semester was a disaster. Academically, neither one of us did anything. I remember faithfully going to Psychology 103, but that's it. At the time, I had an engineering major and didn't want to be an engineer anymore. I didn't go to any of those classes.

To the average person, nothing was wrong. I appeared to be taking care of business, but that couldn't have been further from the truth. Socially, I was having a ball. I was hitting the club every Thursday for College Night. Nobody, not even me, knew what was going on. Upon reflection, I know that something was wrong.

What's going on today is not too different. I am not taking care of business. I am functioning at a higher level now than I was then. When people think of depression, they tend to think the depressed person is walking around sad and blue. At no point have I been sad. I feel like my spirits have been pretty high considering what I I've been dealing with. I would think I would know if I was sad, considering the amount of time I spend alone. I am happy.

An allegory...

I woke up in a hole. The last thing I remember is walking up a steep hill. I had been walking up that hill for some time. No one I knew had made that climb before, but I bravely put on my gear and started walking. I wasn't alone for much of my climb. There were people cheering me on along the way as if it were a race. One person even walked with me for a while. But this journey was mine. Inevitably, I had to take it alone.

There was a hole. It was pitch black in this hole. I didn't feel panic though. I just didn't know where I was and how I got there. God has always afforded me the ability to stay calm in strange situations. I wandered around in the dark for a while trying to find my way. Nothing. It was like being blind. I huddled in a corner. Defeated. For days I sat there...in the dark...starved. Starved for food, human contact, and sunlight.

In those days in the darkness, I had lost touch with myself, my spirituality. I was decaying inside. The game is different down here. You do what you have to do to survive. Already emotionally spent from the trip up the hill, how was I now supposed to deal with being in this hole? I was starting to lose my mind.

Those moments in the dark were unpleasant because I'm not a big fan of the unknown. I had to figure out a way to get out of this hole. My fight was starting to kick in. Something I was unable to see before appeared to me...a sliver of light. It was shining from above through the hole. That small beam of light gave me hope. I was now determined to get out of this hole.

To be continued....

Part 2: The Saga Continues

4.07.09

Nipples

S	M	T	W	T	F	S
			1	2	3	4
5	6	7	8	9	10	11
12	13	14	15	16	17	18
19	20	21	22	23	24	25
26	27	28	29	30		

April 2009

Medications: None

Treatments: Nipple Creation

Today I got my nipples. No areolas, but just nipples. It was an in-office procedure. My mother insisted that she come along to see it. I had fully adjusted to having no nipples and wasn't particularly excited about getting some after all this time. I polled quite a few people as to whether they thought I should get nipples. Many of the people I talked to, mostly men, said to get them. The rationale was that in the long run, I probably didn't want to have to explain why I didn't have any nipples.

The procedure was fairly simple and quick. He was going to use my own skin to make the nipples. He numbed the area via injection. He cut 2 diamond shaped sections of skin and a small round flap. I didn't watch, but somehow he twisted the skin around to form a nipple. What I didn't like was the sound of the scissors as he cut the skin. Sometimes listening to the procedure was worse than watching the procedure. If you have an active imagination like I do, then the images that pop-up in your head can be pretty bad.

I had to stay bandaged for a few days. I drove my mother home that same day. I was numbed up pretty well. In the past, I have always had my mother change my bandages because I don't do blood. I had taken my mother back home though, so I had to do some of it.

6.02.09

Areolas

	JUNE 2009					
S	M	T	W	T	F	S
	1	2	3	4	5	6
7	8	9	10	11	12	13
14	15	16	17	18	19	20
21	22	23	24	25	26	27
28	29	30				

Medications: None

Treatments: Areola Creation

Today I got my areolas. That's all.

Erica J
06/03/09

So I write...
To clear my head
To clear my mind
It's a mess in there
It'll all be fine
I tell myself
Not quite convinced
It seems I've gone and
Lost my way
Lord...help...me
I pray
Just
Slow
It
Down
To figure it out
The answers will come
And relieve my doubt

So I write...
As therapy
There are so many issues
Bothering me
My words
Soothing
They comfort me

Eventually
I'll get this Ph.D
On some days
I'm not so sure
Because I'm still dealing
With this cancer
I wonder
What's in store for me
...............................struggling to finish this poem

Erica was grateful for the care she received from loved ones – one in particular...

Please discuss the ways in which the nominee has cared for a person or people dealing with cancer. (600 words or less).

I was diagnosed with Stage 1 Breast Cancer in October 2007 at the age of 31. At the time, I was in Louisville, KY working on my doctoral degree. She was in Cincinnati, OH. For much of my life it's pretty much been she and I. My mother and I are like best friends. When I was diagnosed, it broke her heart and on top of that I was living in a different city so she felt she would be limited on how she could help me.

I did not have a support system in Louisville to assist me with going to and from chemotherapy treatments and the various surgeries I needed to have. My mother essentially relocated from Cincinnati to Louisville to help me. Between October 2007 and April 2009 my mother made her way down from Cincinnati to take care of me during my lumpectomy, fertility preservation surgery, each of the six rounds of chemotherapy, double mastectomy and reconstruction, nipple reconstruction, and medical tattooing.

When she found out that I had breast cancer and how much it was going to cost, she didn't skip a beat. As a full-time graduate student, I didn't have a significant income and only had student health insurance. She coordinated a raffle that would help raise money to pay for my treatments and surgeries.

There is no way I could possibly repay her for the time she spent nursing me back to physical health following my surgeries and chemotherapy treatments. She prepared my meals. She fed me. She bathed me. She clothed me. She changed my drains even when it made her sick. She drove me back and forth in a city that was unfamiliar to her.

I am completely in her debt for nursing me back to emotional health. She was a one woman cheerleading squad. She was there when I cut off all my hair. She was there when I bought my wigs. She was the one who encouraged me to continue to go to class when I didn't feel like going. And when all of the surgeries were done and I was in remission, she was the one who noticed I was suffering from depression. She helped me to cope with was the most trying situation I had ever encountered in my 31 years of life.

I am grateful to the woman who has always been my support system. I hope that you consider my mother for this award for all of the great things she has done for me.

Thank you for submitting your nomination for the Vitas Caregiver Award!

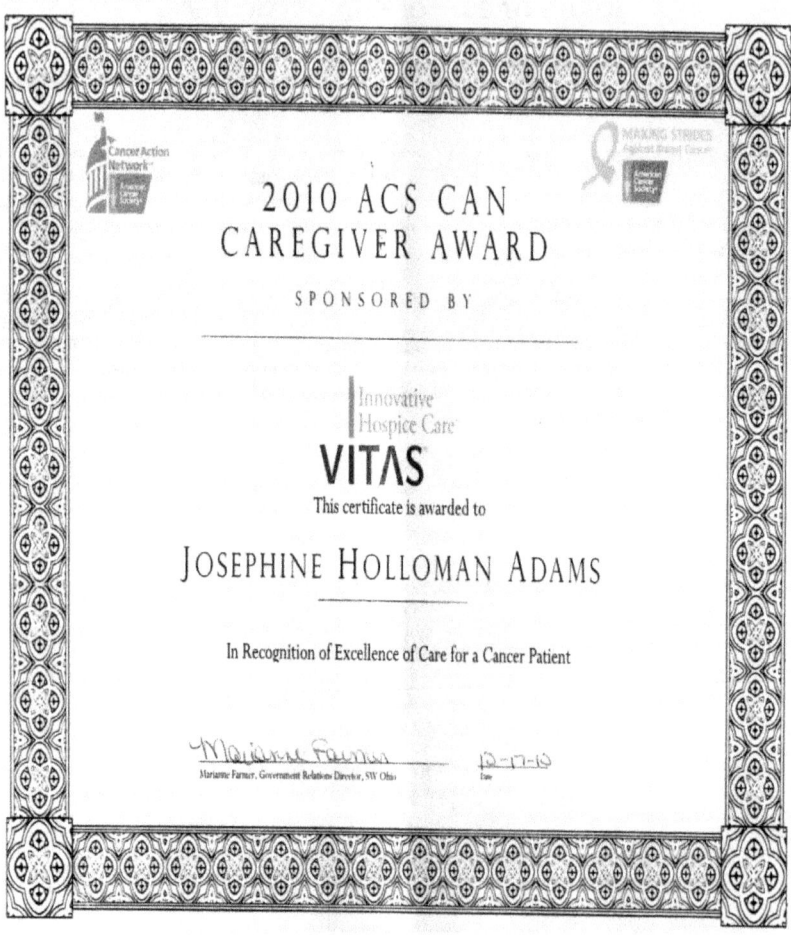

Part 3:
The Fertility Files

"I've finally found someone who is willing to face my future fertility challenges with me. Chemotherapy tried to rob me of my ability to have children."

This part of the book originally began as The Fertility Files. This was supposed to be my journey to having a child. Little did I know that the dream would be thwarted...

5.12.10

Another Consult

	MAY 2010					
S	M	T	W	T	F	S
						1
2	3	4	5	6	7	8
9	10	11	12	13	14	15
16	17	18	19	20	21	22
23	24	25	26	27	28	29
30	31					

Medications: None

Treatments: Fertility Consult

The oncologist referred me an infertility doctor associated with Wake Forest Baptist. I wanted to consult with the doctor to find out my chances of having a baby...

09.10

The Doctor

	SEPTEMBER 2010					
S	M	T	W	T	F	S
			1	2	3	4
5	6	7	8	9	10	11
12	13	14	15	16	17	18
19	20	21	22	23	24	25
26	27	28	29	30		

Medications: None

Treatments: Semen Analysis

McKenzie (prayerfully my future baby's daddy) and I had an 11:00 a.m. appointment for him to give a semen sample. We walked into the doctor's office and there were several couples waiting. We filled out the appropriate paperwork and paid the $120 for the lab work. The doctor called back that afternoon. They had done a semen analysis.

10.06.10

Returns

	October 2010					
S	M	T	W	T	F	S
					1	2
3	4	5	6	7	8	9
10	11	12	13	14	15	16
17	18	19	20	21	22	23
24	25	26	27	28	29	30
31						

Medications: None

Treatments: Semen Analysis

He had to go back to the clinic to give a 2nd sample...

10.23.10

Menses

S	M	T	W	T	F	S
					1	2
3	4	5	6	7	8	9
10	11	12	13	14	15	16
17	18	19	20	21	22	23
24	25	26	27	28	29	30
31						

October 2010

Medications: Clomid

Treatments: None

I came on my period...as scheduled. Completely disappointing. I had taken the Clomid as prescribed. We thought trying naturally would work. We had sex for six days straight. Most of those days it was twice per day during the time when I thought I would be ovulating.

11.06.10

The Big Day!!

NOVEMBER 2010

S	M	T	W	T	F	S
	1	2	3	4	5	6
7	8	9	10	11	12	13
14	15	16	17	18	19	20
21	22	23	24	25	26	27
28	29	30				

Medications: Tylenol, Clomid, Ovidrel, Femara

Treatments: Insemination, IVF

Today's the big day! I get inseminated. My appointment is at 9:30 a.m. I've endured a lot of pain to get to this day. I can only pray that it works...

I arrive at the doctor's office a little early. When I arrive, I am told that my sample is ready and that I could go into the room. Before I went into the room I went to get a cup of water so I could take some Tylenol. I was told that there may be some mild cramping.

I walked into the room and undressed from the waist down. No sooner than I sat down did Dr. Y walk in. He briefed me on the situation. We talked about my egg reserve which was in the normal range, but on the low end. We also talked about sperm counts. A good range is between 1 and 5 million sperm. Immediately my mind started wandering. The process is to freeze, thaw, and then wash the sperm. What happens if his count is low? Can I handle him going to a doctor because of me? What if.....? Erica stop, just stop! Urg.

He also suggested that in-vitro fertilization (IVF) might have better success since my egg reserve isn't as high. Nevertheless, we were going to go ahead with this procedure anyway. It only takes one, right?

With my feet in stirrups, he elevated my chair. He then inserted a catheter directly into my uterus to deposit the semen. There was some mild cramping associated with this, but it was manageable. I had to lie back in that position for 10 minutes.

After getting dressed, I sought out the doctor. I needed to ask him questions about Clomid. I informed him that the Clomid was causing me incredible back pain. I also told him that after I took the Ovidrel shot, when I woke up the next morning it felt like someone had kicked me in the ribs. He was shocked to find out that the drugs had those side effects. He said that he could prescribe something else, like Femara. I told him that I had taken Femara before. He asked why there was a switch. I didn't know, but I know I didn't have seriously debilitating side effects with it. As for the Ovidrel side effects he informed me that was painful ovulation and there was nothing that could be done about that.

Next steps: Wait to see whether I come on my period or not. If I don't come on my period, then I should take a home pregnancy test. If I do, then we'll start this process all over again...with Femara.

11.30.10

Old Tricks

	NOVEMBER 2010					
S	M	T	W	T	F	S
	1	2	3	4	5	6
7	8	9	10	11	12	13
14	15	16	17	18	19	20
21	22	23	24	25	26	27
28	29	30				

Medications: None

Treatments: Gastroenterologist Visit

Well...Cancer's back up to its old tricks.

I had an appointment with the gastroenterologist today...

12.01.10

Hospital

S	M	T	W	T	F	S
			1	2	3	4
5	6	7	8	9	10	11
12	13	14	15	16	17	18
19	20	21	22	23	24	25
26	27	28	29	30	31	

December 2010

Medications: None

Treatments: Hospital Stay

My sleep was uncomfortable in that hospital bed.

During the night, my aunts and my parents arrived.

My mother spent the night.

12.09.10

More...

December 2010						
S	M	T	W	T	F	S
			1	2	3	4
5	6	7	8	9	10	11
12	13	14	15	16	17	18
19	20	21	22	23	24	25
26	27	28	29	30	31	

Medications: None

Treatments: Chemotherapy

Chemo I

12.31.10

Macy's

	DECEMBER 2010					
S	M	T	W	T	F	S
			1	2	3	4
5	6	7	8	9	10	11
12	13	14	15	16	17	18
19	20	21	22	23	24	25
26	27	28	29	30	31	

Medications: None

Treatments: None

I decided to go downtown to Macy's with my parents and McKenzie. We had a few items to return.

While in the store, my head got hot. I had not put a wig on. I put on the hat that Bobby gave me.

My mother suggested that I should just take my hat off. I thought about it for a moment.

Taking the hat off would be a big move for me. Up until this point, I had only worn my bald head in the house around friends and family.

1.03.11

Chemo

JANUARY 2011						
S	M	T	W	T	F	S
						1
2	3	4	5	6	7	8
9	10	11	12	13	14	15
16	17	18	19	20	21	22
23	24	25	26	27	28	29
30	31					

Medications: None

Treatments: Chemotherapy

Today is Chemo #2. I can't say that I'm excited because I truly don't know what to expect. The last chemo was under the influence of a variety of meds. This chemo will determine how the rest of them go.

8:45 a.m. - I have labs today, then I meet with the doctor, and then I have chemo. I'm thinking about going to work tomorrow for a few hours.

1.04.11

Wash Day

S	M	T	W	T	F	S
						1
2	3	4	5	6	7	8
9	10	11	12	13	14	15
16	17	18	19	20	21	22
23	24	25	26	27	28	29
30	31					

January 2011

Medications: Neulasta

Treatments: None

Today, I washed my hair.

I'm still feeling nauseous.

My mother is sick.

Went to work today for three hours

Doctor's appointment for Neulasta

A taste in my mouth that I can't get rid of

1.06.11

The Easy Part

	JANUARY 2011					
S	M	T	W	T	F	S
						1
2	3	4	5	6	7	8
9	10	11	12	13	14	15
16	17	18	19	20	21	22
23	24	25	26	27	28	29
30	31					

Medications: None

Treatments: None

...sometimes dealing with the disease is the easy part. This is how I'm feeling after talking to McKenzie today. He feels as if I don't take his feelings into consideration in reference to what I'm going through. This cancer is trying to kill me. I'll be on this planet as long as it takes to serve my purpose...whatever that is. I try not to get bogged down with the thought that one day the cancer will overtake my body. I want to live. I want a high quality of life. I want to have children and I want to be here to see them as adults. I hope that God can hear my pleas and my prayers.

How to stay positive....Helping your partner deal.

1.20.11 – 3.31.11

January
February
March
2011

Medications: None

Treatments: PET scan, Chemotherapy

January 20, 2011

My husband (Bobby) and some friends from home came to celebrate Erica's birthday. She had a really good weekend. I needed to see him even though I watched her every move. We went to a game and had dinner and cake at my nieces house.

January 21: Erica had a PET scan. We all went to the hospital for the scan.

January 22, 2011: HAPPY 35th Birthday ERICA!!!

January 23, 2011: Bobby back home. Missing him already.

January 24, 2011: The doctor called. He said after two chemo treatments you can barely see anything in the bones, shoulders or pelvis. The nodes in the liver are much smaller. Not only do the results look good they "LOOK GREAT." We are very happy.

February 2011

We both agree that her body is not popping back from this chemo like it did the last time.

March 17, 2011

After labs today I get to go home. Labs don't go so well. Her blood count was low. She was told to rest and stay away from people. Should I go? Not sure now. Do I trust someone else with her care? She insisted I go. I was worried the whole time. Erica is going to a conference and her friends assured me they would take care of her. She assures me she will use the handicap route, wheelchairs, etc. I return one day earlier than her.

March 30, 2011: Erica returns from conference

March 31, 2011: CHEMO

3.31.11

Chemo

S	M	T	W	T	F	S
		1	2	3	4	5
6	7	8	9	10	11	12
13	14	15	16	17	18	19
20	21	22	23	24	25	26
27	28	29	30	31		

MARCH 2011

Medications: None

Treatments: Chemotherapy

March 31, 2011
Chemo

4.07.11

Scan

	APRIL 2011					
S	M	T	W	T	F	S
					1	2
3	4	5	6	7	8	9
10	11	12	13	14	15	16
17	18	19	20	21	22	23
24	25	26	27	28	29	30

Medications: None

Treatments: PET Scan

April 7, 2011

PET Scan today. Pray for a clean scan!

4.11.11 – 4.12.11

Results

	APRIL 2011					
S	M	T	W	T	F	S
					1	2
3	4	5	6	7	8	9
10	11	12	13	14	15	16
17	18	19	20	21	22	23
24	25	26	27	28	29	30

Medications: None

Treatments: PET Scan Results

April 11, 2011
I'm officially in REMISSION, bay-bee!!! Praise Him! Thanks for all the positive thoughts and prayers!

> *April 11, 2011: REMISSION!!! Come back in 3 months for another scan. YES! We made it!!!*

April 12, 2011
McKenzie said, "Good Morning Beautiful! Day2 of Remission! Amen Again!! 2500!!"

> *April 12, 2011: ERICA is a 2x survivor 2011*

5.11

From Mama

		MAY 2011				
S	M	T	W	T	F	S
1	2	3	4	5	6	7
8	9	10	11	12	13	14
15	16	17	18	19	20	21
22	23	24	25	26	27	28
29	30	31				

Medications: None

Treatments: None

I did not want to leave, but Erica was cancer free and she wanted me to leave so that both of us could kind of get back to a normal life. Her scans were both cancer free, so I thought it was ok because she was so insistent.

It had been 6 months and I had visited home twice. When I reached Greensboro Airport, I felt funny. I did not want to leave but she was like, "no you need to go." When I got home, I could not put my finger on this feeling but I told my husband, pastor and my sister that the only word I could come up with was "TROUBLED." I said, "I am troubled and I don't know why" I felt this way for a month.

6.03.11

Results Are In

		JUNE 2011				
S	M	T	W	T	F	S
			1	2	3	4
5	6	7	8	9	10	11
12	13	14	15	16	17	18
19	20	21	22	23	24	25
26	27	28	29	30		

Medications: None

Treatments: Radiation Therapy

Results are in. I've gotta do radiation therapy. There are two spots on my spine that chemo didn't get. Ideally, it will help solve this pain problem I've been having. I start next week. Anything that's gonna help solve this pain is welcomed. It's not bad news...it's just news.

6.04.11

No Pain, All Gain

S	M	T	W	T	F	S
			1	2	3	4
5	6	7	8	9	10	11
12	13	14	15	16	17	18
19	20	21	22	23	24	25
26	27	28	29	30		

June 2011

Medications: None

Treatments: None

I woke up pain free this morning! Hallelujah! I'll take it for as long as I can get it...

6.11

Rapid Fire

JUNE 2011

S	M	T	W	T	F	S
			1	2	3	4
5	6	7	8	9	10	11
12	13	14	15	16	17	18
19	20	21	22	23	24	25
26	27	28	29	30		

Medications: Pain Medicine, 'The Shot'

Treatments: Radiation, Hospital Stay

Wednesday, June 8, 2011

10:00 a.m. First radiation for Erica. She called me and was happy and said radiation was over. I asked her if she was going to work or home. She said she was going to work. I had been worried all morning.

By 2:00 p.m. Erica decided to leave work because she started to feel sick. She called some time later after she had arrived home stating that on the way home she had the most excruciating pain she had ever felt in her life! She felt pain in her legs. Sick all night. I was scared. I did not tell her. I called my niece and we both kept calling the doctor. This was the start of the change of the rest of my life!

Thursday, June 9, 2011

My niece took Erica to the hospital. She was tired but, talking. I sat by the phone waiting and worried.

Friday, June 10, 2011

Co-worker took her to the hospital. Gina met them there when she arrived Erica was in a wheel chair with a garbage can in her lap because of the nausea. She was very weak and they said dehydrated. Her doctor said, "Erica, I know you are going to hate me but I think we should admit you and get your pain and dehydration under control." Erica said she would stay, "but how long?" He said he would release her on Monday if she was feeling better. Erica really did not want to stay because she said she was going to "A Taste of Charlotte" in Charlotte, North Carolina about an hour away. She was mad. But stayed. LOL. Erica has been admitted to the hospital, tired but talking and texting. I wanted to return to Winston but she said, "no."

Saturday, June 11, 2011

Erica was in the hospital replying only by texting. I'm going. I made a flight to arrive Monday at 4:00 p.m.

Sunday, June 12, 2011

Tired, no talking.

June 13, 2011

7:30 a.m. I am preparing to go to my doctor's appointment. The phone rings. I look at the number; it is from the Hospital.

Me: Hello? (The voice on the other end is the Oncologist)
Doctor: Is this Josie?
Me: Yes.
Doctor: Your daughter is very sick. You need to get here. (It was something in his voice)
Me: Does my husband need to come?
Doctor: Yes, she is very sick. I'M SORRY.

Hum, I cried. I called my sister and she made plans for my husband to be on the flight at 4:00 p.m. I went to my doctor's appointment. What else was I supposed to do?! I already knew.

4:00 p.m. the plane landed. I called her boss and asked if they knew Erica was in the hospital and she said no because they had just saw her and figured she was working from home.

She almost beat me to the hospital. At the hospital by 5:00 p.m. My husband thought that when we got there she would hear our voices and that would be enough for her to pull through this. He just did not know.

When I walked in I knew. I immediately asked for pain medicine because Erica was moaning. I knew she heard me because I asked her several times to open her eyes. When she did I wish I had not. They were so yellow and unfocused, I knew she could not see me. I moved to the other side of the bed and called her name again. "ERICA!' I said "I'm over here". She did not turn in my direction. I started checking her body for signs of....dying. I was also asking questions as she would have done. Not feeling, just doing. My husband and I spent the night taking turns talking to her all night.

June 14, 2011

7:00 a.m. The doctor sat in front of me. He kneeled down and said, "I don't know what happened. I'm sorry."

I cried. My husband sat in the chair in the corner of the room. Before he left he said, "you know it was cancer related don't you." I just looked at him. I thought you said you did not know what happened.

The doctor said "You should call your family if they want to get here". He said "I'm sorry". Without thinking I knew my life would never be the same. I called my niece and her husband and told her what the doctor said. Erica only had days or a week to live. Erica was still mumbling to questions asked of her but not opening her eyes. Our pastor from home called and Erica actually sat up and opened her eyes looking around for him. She listened and responded accordingly.

I sat by her side the rest of the day. At first I did not want any friends and only a few family members around but the doctor said let them all come, let her hear their voices. That afternoon they did come. I know it was many because I was there but I was still trying to control the situation.

I stepped into Erica mode. My family, her best friend, her boyfriend, and friends from work and Charlotte came. While they were there the nurse came in and said WOW she is really a fighter and from nowhere Erica said, "um hum" real loud. That told us she could hear us. We all laughed. She was controlling the situation. We spent the night again.

About 4:00 a.m. the nurse came in and said the signs were there that Erica was transitioning. Was I ready for the shot? How do I answer that? Am I ready to let go? Am I ready to never see my daughter again??

Am……I……ready?

We said yes and cried. (Her mom, her dad, and her boyfriend).

6:40 a.m. I called my family and told them the doctor said if they want to see her for the last time they needed to get back. We *cried and I said yes. I held Erica in my arms - no life. I hope she knew.*

June 15, 2011

7:54 a.m. ERICA died. I'm so sad! I hope she felt me...LOVE HER TO THE END!!

They told me to push to help get her into the world. I told them to push to help her leave this world. It's like the old saying, "I brought you into this world and I will take you out". Not suffering anymore, cancer not going to her brain, this helps comfort me. She was worried about cancer going to her brain and what her quality of life would be. Now she does not have to worry. I won't have to look in or at her eyes helpless. Neither one of us not being able to control or change what the outcome might be. Does she know, will she remember?

The day my life changed/ended was not June 15, 2011 the day Erica died. It was June 13, 2011 the day he doctor called. That's the day I knew her life was ending. Somehow I knew things started changing for me then. The 15th of June finalized what I knew at that moment at 7:00 a.m. on June 13, 2011. I started living with a broken heart.

June 16, 2011

Erica's Body arrives home, Cincinnati, OHIO

Mortality

I don't wanna think about that which I know to be true

Death is Coming

It's coming for each one of us

Our time is not our own

Growing older

Day after Day

Brings us closer to that moment in which life ceases to exist

I can't bear to watch my loved ones die

One by One

Truth is...

Life is death

Death is life

(Written by Erica J. Holloman, August 2007)

Was I Really Dreaming

June 23, 2011

Dreaming: I was sitting in the balcony looking down at the funeral as it was happening, as if I was looking through someone else eyes watching myself shut the casket. I saw me and Bobby standing to the side waiting for the family to finish viewing the body when they all sit down and the song "If I could" by Regina Belle started playing. I saw Bobby and I walk over to the casket to view Erica's body.

I watched myself (I'm looking at the back of myself work). I saw myself look at her for a minute, then I watched as I tucked her in for the last time. I watched me fold the lining of her casket down folding carefully around her head, arms and waist. I saw me turn to the funeral director so he could take the light off the top of the casket. I saw him reposition the book we had in her casket (because if you knew Erica you knew she always had a book in her hands). I watched him remove the special piece I had embroidered with her name and sorority chapter on it. I watched him fold it and set it aside. I watched him step aside then I saw myself look and when I knew she was carefully tucked in, I saw me carefully close the top to put her to rest forever.

I watched myself move to the bottom of the casket to crank and lock the casket. I watched me almost trip over Bobby getting back to the head of the casket to touch it as I wept. While watching Bobby put the cap over the lock. I was handed the crank to keep. I watched him and myself just standing and looking at the casket. Just looking. I am looking at my back, I see the back of my hair, that slight flip that I only see in the mirror. I know what the back of my suit looks like. I clearly see the back of my legs, the sheer off black stockings, the hills of my black pumps only once slightly seeing the silhouette of my face as if I was looking through someone else's eyes. Or as if someone or something allowed me to see this part of my daughter's funeral. Then I watched as we sat down.

I was allowed to experience the exact, same thing June 24, 2011. How could I have seen that?

Fertility Revisited

Lots of people knew about the embryos, but few people knew Bobby and I had come to the decision to use them. I had intentionally put the decision of using them or even dealing with them in the back of my mind. Subconsciously I knew they were there but acted like I did not have another thing to deal with.

Bobby and I sat down and decided that since we told Erica we would take care of her children if something happened to her we decided we would use her embryos. But first we had to see if they really belonged to us. He also said he did not want many people to know because this would be our decision. HE did not want to hear anyone's opinion. He did not care what people had to say because this was our business. Until this moment most people did not know.

8-2012 – I decided to call the fertility doctor that Erica had in Winston-Salem to get her advice as well as some education about IVF. I informed her that I was thinking about using the embryos and had made an appointment with the fertility doctor in Louisville where the embryos were frozen and in storage. She said she knows him and he was a good doctor. She explained what could possibly happen using a surrogate. How much it could cost. And what the percentages were for success. She wanted me to keep her informed and told me I could call her back if I had questions and wished me luck. I felt better after speaking with her.

9/2012 - First Meeting with the fertility doctor in Louisville Ky. Are the Embryo's mine?

I knew legally the embryo's belonged to me, but did they as far as the doctor was concerned? I have not really thought this through but I wanted to know what if? I had briefly explained the situation to the doctor over the phone so when we sat in his office for the first visit he was caught up on the situation. He remembered Erica.

He explained that the perfect age for a gestational carrier was between the ages of 22 to 32. Has had a least one child, and they prefer she be a cousin, *friend or family member, only because she is more likely to give you the child without problems.*

With a smile on his face he wanted to know "what is your plan"? Humm….. He explained he had successfully inseminated a woman my age. As if I was going to do it! My husband had already said no to that. He explained the chance of success and failure. He said he could make it happen because the embryos were my property. He stated that when someone dies they usually look for the next of kin. I would need to send court papers showing ownership.

-1-

There are 3 embryos and since the father is a donor there would be no legal fight with another parent. He also said a carrier could cost anywhere from $25,000 to $35,000 and usually and IVF agency charges $5,000 to $7,000 up charge. He explained that the delivering woman is considered legally the mother; therefore you must have legal papers drawn up before the process begins. I could come to him in Louisville for the procedures or he could send the embryos to Cincinnati. But he wanted to see this thru.

He also explained the mapping procedure, where they go in and map out the exact place they will be insemination.

He asked if we had any questions.

Q. Do very many Black women volunteer to carry babies for other people?
A. No, not many.

Q. Will a White woman carry a Black baby?
A. Sometimes...maybe

He felt we fell into a category where people may understand our plight or someone may feel sorry for us so they may do it. And remember we would also be paying for a service. Paying someone to carry our baby.

At this time we did not have any idea what we were in store for, but we decided not to move the embryo's to Cincinnati because I trusted the doctor and moving them also has a cost associated with it. The laws were different in Ohio and Kentucky. Ohio is actually more lenient with surrogacy laws than KY. In KY surrogacy is illegal but you can have a gestational carrier. But the main reason I wanted them to stay there was because the doctor knew Erica and was familiar with the case.

Sept/Oct 2012 – I had been explaining the process to a close friend explaining surrogacy and just what I was thinking and or planning. Shortly after we hung up I received a phone call.

She was crying. She said that someone I knew wanted to volunteer to carry the baby for Erica. I was silent could not speak. I said "she would do that for me"? She said I think she is doing it for Erica. I had never had a conversation about this with this person. I never imagined someone would do something so beautiful and selfless for me. What would make her do this?

It was a few days before I called her.

-2-

The Volunteer

27 years old, African American, Single mom does not smoke, drink, or do drugs. HEALTHY. Works, drives, no significant other. Has known Erica her whole life. Perfect Fit.

11-8-12 Fertility Doctor – We were told that the Gestational Carries would have to have someone with her to represent her best interest. To make sure we were not forcing her into this. On the way to pick her up I was nervous. As we drove to get her I was thinking all kind of things. What if she changes her mind? What if the doctor says she can't do it? What if? I was nervous all the way to Louisville.

11-29-12 I spoke with an attorney today about handling our case. I feel like I'm standing still not moving.

12-7-12 Office visit with attorney – Her office was full of things, books, paintings, but charming. I felt warm, comfortable like being in someone's house. I wondered what she thought of us sitting on the other side of the desk considering being parents at our age.

She had not handled very many surrogate cases and none like this. She explained the child must be born in Hamilton County, no travel for the surrogate after she reached a certain stage because if the child was born out of town it could be a problem. She also explained that both parties would have to have their own attorney for the safety of all involved. We learned that the woman carrying the baby was considered the birth mother and that we would have to adopt our own baby!

12-10-12 Psychologist visits both parties involved; as part of the process we had to have a psychological evaluation before we went any further. They needed to make sure we were, I guess, going to be good parents and not crazy. Also to makes sure our Gestational Carrier would be ok with giving the baby to us once it was born and be able to walk away. Also to make sure we were not forcing her to do this. Oh and to make sure she was not crazy! OK people really, this whole process is crazy! Just the thought of what we are doing is just crazy.

EVALUATION: The Adams and their gestational carrier, no emotional illness. You may proceed.

The psychologist suggested to the carrier a few books that would help explain to her child that she was doing us a favor by carrying the baby for us and they can come visit anytime they wanted to.

-3-

4-9-13 Fertility Doctor Louisville KY – Some days this ride back and forth to Louisville KY is hard so I asked if some of the procedures could be done in Cincinnati. The doctor agreed. Yes. The blood work, ultra sounds and pregnancy test could be done in Cincinnati.

4-24-13 We met early in the morning at a lab in Cincinnati before she was to report to work for labs, but after she dropped her child off to school. I arrived early, waiting, thinking, would she come, should I call her? Relief she's here. As usual I handled all the paper work, set up future appointments then waited while she went back for blood work and ultrasound. I always had a smile when she came out we would walk to the parking lot together she went her way I went mine. Then I waited for the Doctors office in Louisville to call the next day with the results.

5-2-13 8:00 a.m. Ultra Sound/Blood work Cincinnati

5-6-13 8:00 a.m. Ultra Sound/Blood work Cincinnati

6-4-13 we have to be in Louisville at 11:00am don't forget to bring water because she has to have a full bladder. Measure the uterus (Mapping)

6-8-13 start Progesterone

6-10-13 today is Monday. Tomorrow is the day we go to see the fertility doctor for the insemination. One way or the other, our lives will never be the same.

We were running errands. I looked up and saw my church. I asked Bobby if we could go in and have the pastor pray for us. It was not the first time I asked him. He always said no. But this time he said yes. There were many occasions when I came close to telling the pastor what we were planning. I wanted him to just listen, not judge, not read me scripture - just pray for my soul. I went to the secretary's office to ask if we could speak to the pastor. She said he's off today. My heart hit the floor. My soul silently cried a river. I needed somebody to pray for me! I was like, 'he gets an off day?' I laughed. She said you can come back tomorrow. I went back to the car and told Bobby he was off today. Silence. He said what do you want to do? I said, 'go home. Come back tomorrow.' I needed prayer now not tomorrow,

tomorrow would be too late. I would be on my way to Louisville.

6-11-13 Full Bladder, Insemination Day, - I was going to wait in a chair outside the IVF room but the nurse said I should go in. She said most people wanted to be there when the procedure took place. She said just be there. I was glad I did. The IVF room was small, beige, with lots of instruments all around. The bed was in the center of the room with a portable ultra sound machine. There was an adjoining room witch held the thawed embryos. It's a secret room only select people go into it.

<u>1:07pm WE ARE PRENGANT!</u>

-4-

The doctor wanted us to stay in Louisville overnight. We booked a hotel about 7 miles away. Checking in, I know the people behind the desk just thought we were like any other travelers getting 2 adjoining rooms. They had no way of knowing she had just done something so amazing, overwhelming and selfless. Not only for her dead friend but a mother silently hoping for a chance to hold her daughters baby in her arms and be allowed to love someone unconditionally again. I will never forget the kindness and love she showed me. I wanted to hold her in my arms and let her feel how much I loved her at the moment, while at the same time holding back, respecting the relationship we always had. I worried all night knowing she was in the adjacent room. The door was slightly open and I listened for her every movement. Did she need help? How was she feeling? Did the transfer work? Keep your legs propped up on the pillow! Silently worrying in the adjacent rooms.

6-12-13 8:30am Pregnancy Test- Cincinnati Ohio

6-24-13 - My heart is saddened again today. I guess like so many women who tried IVF and are told that the results are negative I am again crushed. I knew it was only a 35 percent chance but I so wanted it to work. To see a part of my daughter's seed, her spirit, maybe even her eyes.

Until recently I did not ever allow myself to think past the fact that the embryos were just that embryos. I never looked at baby things nor did I plan on buying anything until the day he/she came home. I did not attach onto the fact that I would be a mother again or the fact that for the first time someone would call me mommy.

At 2:22pm June 24th I received a call from the IVF nurse in Louisville saying she had bad news.

"It did not work". The TEST was NEGATIVE!!! "I'm SORRY". There were those words again - "I'm sorry". I could hear tears in her voice. She said that my carrier should stop taking all med's. My response was... ok.

After a couple of minutes I started to cry. The fertility nurse wanted to know if I wanted her to call my Gestational carrier, I was not sure. How do you tell someone who has selflessly given her life, time and dreams to you for a whole year that all the shots, blood draws, urine test, and the ultra sounds led to SORRY it did not work.

Bobby asked what she said. I told him through tears what she had said and it was as if he froze in time. He simply dropped his head trying to hide his tears. He said "I am so disappointed. I just knew it would work. What happened?" I reminded him it was a 35 percent chance. He continued to shake his head.

-5-

Just when I thought I was no different than a lot of women who go through IVF, I suddenly realized I was. I have been walking in my daughters footsteps. I was the one to see the picture of the ultra sound, I was the one to speak up for her unborn embryos, and I was the one to feel the pain of not reaching motherhood. This is where I am like other mothers. I am glad it was me who experienced this pain and not Erica. I did everything I could so that my daughter could be a mother. I could not have lived knowing she would feel this pain of not becoming a mother. Better me than her.

I called my gestational carrier at 2:32pm she said she was ok.

6-24-13 - 4:05pm the fertility doctor called he said "stop taking meds, no other appointment needed"

Shortly after I heard a knock on the door it was my carrier. We held each other and cried for a while she could not believe it did not work. We did everything we were supposed to do. I said, "I know". I did not talk to anyone for 3 weeks. I just did not have anything to say.

UPDATES

Four things Erica wanted to do that her father and I are following through with:

1. The *Erica J. Holloman Bra Drive* was started by Erica before she died. The first year she donated 70 bras. The second year she donated over 500 bras. To date, with the help of our community, we have donated over 1,500 new bras in Erica's name. The bras are donated to women in Back-To-Work programs, battered women's shelters, and underserved women. This year, for the first time, a gift box with new bras was donated to a woman newly diagnosed with Triple Negative Breast Cancer. Each bra has a hand stitched ribbon saying "Smiling For Erica"

2. *2014 Calendar* featuring survivors and caregivers

3. Before Erica died, she wanted to give me something to say "Thank You". She could not find what she was looking for so she created a line of jewelry to say thank you to all care givers. Her notes were so good that her father has had the line of jewelry created and has an online store selling the jewelry to honor caregivers. Our web store is called "CareGiver Thank You!"

4. If you are reading this, this is the fourth thing on her list. She wrote this book. She told her story. And we followed through.

All of these products can be found at
www.ericajhollomanfoundationinc.org

Memorial service at Wake Forest September 13, 2011

Proclamation given by the Mayor of Cincinnati declaring October 22, 2011 'Erica Holloman Day' in the City of Cincinnati Ohio

'The Erica J. Holloman Foundation For The Awareness of Triple Negative Breast Cancer' was founded January 22, 2013

University of Louisville gives The Erica J. Holloman Achievement Award annually

The Pi Sigma Zeta Chapter of Zeta Phi Beta Sorority, Inc. (Forest Park Ohio) gives 'The Erica J. Holloman High School Senior Scholarship Award' annually

Wake Forest University gave $1,000 for 'Outstanding Essay' in memory of Erica Holloman. Presented to a student who demonstrated a passion for multicultural education (established April 25, 2013)

On May 9, 2014 the University of Louisville awarded Erica her PhD.

She is official! *Dr. Erica J. Holloman* or

Erica J. Holloman, PhD

Erica is the first in our immediate family to earn the title of doctor. Amen!

Donations consist of lots of things.

WHAT ABOUT BRAS?

Help women in your community

THE 5ᵀᴴ ANNUAL ERICA J. HOLLOMAN Bra Drive

BUY A NEW BRA
(Bras must have purchase tags attached or in original package)
MAIL BRAS TO ADDRESS BELOW

JUNE 15ᵀᴴ – JULY 19ᵀᴴ

We collect NEW BRAS and donate them to women's shelters and other organizations that assist women who are striving to get back to work and start new lives.

Thank You for your support!

SPONSORED BY:

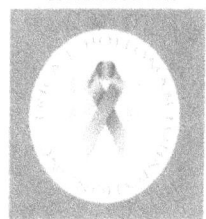

Visit:

www.ericajhollomanfoundationinc.org

Donations can be sent by mail to:

**P.O. Box 14334
Cincinnati, Ohio 45250-0334**

Monetary donations accepted: Bras will be purchased

A LETTER FROM ERICA'S COLLEAGUE:

Hi Mrs. Holloman,

This is Kia Pruitt! It was such an honor meeting you at the awards ceremony where I was honored to receive an award in your daughter's name.

I cannot tell you how honored and blessed I feel to receive such a prestigious award. Without your daughter, MANY of us would not have graduated. Recently, at a dinner with my colleagues and Dr. Cuyjet, Dr. Cuyjet shared with the group that I passed comprehensive exams because Erica had given me notes and stayed on me and made me study. LOL. When he shared my story, every single person around the table said, "That happened to Kia? Wow, Erica did the SAME THING TO ME TOO!" We could not believe it! We were all saying the same thing. Erica had given us all notes and stayed on us ALL, via email, calls and even personal meetings and said, "Come on Black Folks, let's get it together! We WILL pass this test and graduate!"

One of our colleagues asked, so "She asked you all to come together and study so you could all pass?" We laughed and answered, "NO! Erica didn't ASK anything, she TOLD us what to do and we did it!" And we all laughed. And then cried.

She is a beautiful woman, Mrs. Holloman and I KNOW she is looking down on us and guiding us to this day. It is with much pride that I hold the award which your family and UofL so graciously presented to me. Let's please keep in touch.

Until we see each other again, I love you very, very much!

Let's please stay in touch!
Dr. Kia Pruitt

GLOSSARY

Here you will find a list of terms and phrases used in this book which may be unfamiliar to some. Dr. Holloman wrote these definitions out as a way to help you through the book…

Acupuncture (AK-yoo-PUNK-cher) - the technique of inserting thin needles through the skin at specific points on the body to control nausea, vomiting, and other symptoms.

Alopecia (al-oh-PEE-shuh) - The lack or loss of hair from areas of the body where hair is usually found. Alopecia can be a side effect of chemotherapy.

Artificial insemination (AI) - another name for intrauterine insemination but can also refer to placing sperm in a woman's vagina or cervix when she is ovulating. The sperm then travel into the fallopian tubes, where they can fertilize the woman's egg or eggs.

Blood cell count - The number of red blood cells, white blood cells, and platelets in a sample of blood. This is also called a complete blood count (CBC).

Biopsy - Taking a tissue or organ sample to examine it under a microscope

Blanket Of Hope Society – organization based in Louisville, KY which gives pink fleece blankets to women newly diagnosed with cancer

Breast Cancer - Breast cancer is a disease in which abnormal cells in the breast divide and multiply in an uncontrolled fashion. The cells can invade nearby tissue and can spread through the bloodstream and lymphatic system (lymph nodes) to other parts of the body. Breast Cancer is a malignant tumor that develops in the mammary glands. These tumors are primarily located in the upper external half of the breast or in the nipple. They affect the left breast more frequently than the right, although in rare cases they are present in both breasts.

Breast Reconstruction - A plastic surgery procedure in which the shape of the breast is rebuilt. Many women who choose to have preventive mastectomy also decide to have breast reconstruction, either at the time of the mastectomy or at some later time.

Chemotherapy (kee-moh-THAYR-uh-pee) (also called chemo) - Treatment with drugs that kill cancer cells.

Chemo Protection - In the treatment of cancer, chemoprotective agents are drugs which protect healthy tissue from the toxic effects of anticancer drugs

Clomid – Clomifene (INN) or clomiphene (USAN) (trademarked as Androxal, Clomid and Omifin) is a selective estrogen receptor modulator (SERM) that has become the most widely prescribed drug to induce ovulation in the treatment of female infertility. This synthetic drug is available as a white to pale yellow odorless tablet.

Cryobank - A sperm bank, semen bank or cryobank is a facility or enterprise that collects and stores human sperm from sperm donors for use by women who need donor-provided sperm to achieve pregnancy. Sperm donated by the sperm donor is known as donor sperm, and the process for introducing the sperm into the woman is called artificial insemination, which is a form of third party reproduction.

Depression - **Depression** or **depress(ed)** may refer to Biological terms:

- Depression (mood), a state of low mood and aversion to activity
    - Certain mood disorders such as major depressive disorder and dysthymia, that feature depressed mood are commonly referred to as simply *depression*
- Depression (kinesiology), an anatomical term of motion, refers to downward movement, the opposite of elevation
- Depression (physiology), a reduction in a biological variable or the function of an organ
- Central nervous system depression, physiological depression of the central nervous system that can result in loss of consciousness

Diagnosis - Medical diagnosis (often simply termed diagnosis) refers to both the process of attempting to determine or identify a possible disease or disorder (and diagnosis in this sense can also be termed (medical) diagnostic procedure), and to the opinion reached by this process (also being termed (medical) diagnostic opinion). From the point of view of statistics the diagnostic procedure involves classification tests. It is a major component of, for example, the procedure of a doctor's visit.

Donor Sperm - Sperm from a male who isn't a sex partner (as from a sperm bank, friend, or relative) must remain frozen for at least 6 months before it can be used. This is done so that the donor can be tested twice over 6 months to ensure that he does not have any number of infectious diseases, including the human immunodeficiency virus (HIV).[3] Frozen sperm are less effective than fresh sperm.

Eggs - The egg cell (ovum) is the female haploid reproductive cell (gamete) in oogamous organisms. The egg cell is typically not capable of active movement, and it is much larger than the motile sperm cells. When egg and sperm fuse, a diploid cell (the zygote) is formed, which gradually grows into a new organism.

Egg Donation - A woman receives eggs from a donor that are fertilized and implanted once cancer treatment is completed. Donors are women, usually between the ages of 21 and 34, who are willing to provide their eggs to a recipient. They may be anonymous (unknown) or known to the intended parents. Anonymous donors are recruited through egg donation programs or agencies and are not known to the recipient. However, some couples find donors through advertisements. Recipients should be cautious about recruiting donors without the use of an intermediary to screen the donors and should strongly consider seeking legal counsel. Known (also called directed) donors are generally a close friend or relative of the recipient

Egg Extraction - Transvaginal oocyte retrieval (TVOR), also referred to as oocyte retrieval (OCR) or even simply egg collection, is a technique used in in vitro fertilization (IVF) in order to remove oocytes from the ovary of the female, enabling fertilization outside the body.[1] Transvaginal oocyte retrieval is more properly referred to as transvaginal ovum retrieval when the oocytes have matured into ova, as is normally the case in IVF.

Egg Freezing - Human oocyte cryopreservation (egg freezing) is a novel technology in which a woman's eggs (oocytes) are extracted, frozen and stored. Later, when she is ready to become pregnant, the eggs can be thawed, fertilized, and transferred to the uterus as embryos.

Femara – Letrozole (INN, trade name Femara) is an oral non-steroidal aromatase inhibitor for the treatment of hormonally-responsive breast cancer after surgery

Fertility - Fertility is the natural capability to produce offspring. As a measure, "fertility rate" is the number of offspring born per mating pair, individual or population. Fertility differs from fecundity, which is defined as the *potential* for reproduction (influenced by gamete production, fertilization and carrying a pregnancy to term). A lack of fertility is infertility while a lack of fecundity would be called sterility.

Fertility Specialist - Reproductive endocrinology and infertility (REI) is a surgical subspecialty of obstetrics and gynecology that trains physicians in reproductive medicine addressing hormonal functioning as it pertains to reproduction as well as the issue of infertility. While most REI specialists primarily focus on the treatment of infertility, reproductive endocrinologists are trained to also evaluate and treat hormonal dysfunctions in females and males outside of infertility. Reproductive endocrinologists have specialty training in obstetrics and gynecology (ob-gyn) before they undergo sub-specialty training (fellowship) in REI. Reproductive surgery is a related specialty, where a physician in ob-gyn or urology further specializes to operate on anatomical disorders that affect fertility

Hematoma - A collection of blood outside of a blood vessel. It occurs because the wall of a blood vessel wall, artery, vein or capillary, has been damaged and blood has leaked into tissues where it does not belong. The hematoma may be tiny, with just a dot of blood or it can be large and cause significant swelling.

HER2/neu - A gene that carries the genetic code (recipe)for the HER2 protein. HER2 is found on the surface of some normal cells and plays a role in controlling cell growth. Abnormally high amounts of HER2 may be present on the surface of breast cancer cells in one out of four women, mostly due to increased gene-copy number in the nucleus. This causes the cancer cells to grow rapidly.

Hormone Therapy - Treatment with hormones, drugs to interfere with hormone production or hormone action, or the surgical removal of hormone-producing glands. Hormone therapy may cancer cells or slow their growth.

Immature Eggs - An immature ovum is a cell that goes through the process of oogenesis to become an ovum. It can be an oogonium, an oocyte, or an ootid. An oocyte, in turn, can be either primary or secondary, depending on how far it has come in its process of meiosis.

Invasive breast cancer - Invasive breast cancer (also called infiltrating breast cancer) has spread to the normal tissues within or surrounding the breast, or to other parts of the body through the blood and lymph systems.

There are two main types of invasive breast cancer:

- **Invasive ductal carcinoma (IDC):** IDC begins in the milk ducts and accounts for 70 percent or more of invasive breast cancers.
- **Invasive lobular carcinoma (ILC):** ILC begins in the lobules and is more rare. Sometimes, the origin of the tumor may not be known.

Sometimes, breast cancer can be both invasive and noninvasive: some of the cancer cells have grown into normal tissue and some has remained in the ducts or lobules. This type of cancer is treated as an invasive cancer. In some invasive breast cancers, malignant cells may be present in both the ducts and lobues. This type of "mixed tumor" breast cancer is usually treated as ductal carcinoma.

Invasive breast cancer is the most common type of breast cancer among American women. According to the American Cancer Society, 207,090 new cases of invasive breast cancer were diagnosed in women in 2010.

Invasive breast cancer subtypes -

There are also several subtypes of invasive breast cancer, including:

- **Endocrine-sensitive breast cancer:** Breast cancer cells contain measurable amounts of estrogen or progesterone receptors, making the cancer treatable with hormonal therapies
- **HER2-positive breast cancer:** Breast cancer cells contain excess amounts of the HER2 receptor, making the cancer treatable with anti-HER2 targeted therapies
- **Triple-negative breast cancer:** Breast cancer cells do not contain receptors for estrogen, progesterone, or HER2. This type of cancer cannot be treated with hormonal or anti-HER2 therapy, but can be treated with chemotherapy, radiation, and non-HER2 targeted therapy.
- **Inflammatory breast cancer:** Invasive cancer in which there is no lump or tumor.
- **Medullary carcinoma:** A less common type of IDC where the tumor is soft and fleshy (resembling the medulla in the brain).
- **Metaplastic carcinoma:** A rare type of invasive breast cancer where a portion of the tumor cells have changed to a different type of breast cancer (a mixed tumor)
- **Mucinous carcinoma:** A less common type of IDC, the tumors create thick pools of mucin, a main component of saliva.
- **Papillary carcinoma:** A rare type of IDC that forms in distinct lumps with finger-like projections.

- **Tubular carcinoma:** A less common type of IDC made of collections of small, tube-like cells less than 1 cm in diameter.
- **Paget's disease:** Any of the above forms of breast cancer that directly involves the nipple.
- **Male breast cancer:** A rare form of breast cancer, accounting for less than one percent of all breast cancers. Breast cancer in men usually begins as a lump or mass in a man's breast, and is most commonly treated with a mastectomy or lumpectomy.

IVF (in vitro fertilization) - An assisted reproductive technique that involves removing sperm and eggs, fertilizing them in a laboratory, then placing a fertilized egg in the uterus

In Vitro Maturation - the technique of letting ovarian follicles mature in vitro (traditionally done in test-tubes, flasks, petri dishes etc)

Local Anesthesia - any technique to induce the absence of sensation in part of the body,[1] generally for the aim of inducing local analgesia, that is, local insensitivity to pain, although other local senses may be affected as well. It allows patients to undergo surgical and dental procedures with reduced pain and distress. In many situations, such as cesarean section, it is safer and therefore superior to general anesthesia. It is also used for relief of non-surgical pain and to enable diagnosis of the cause of some chronic pain conditions. Anesthetists sometimes combine both general and local anesthesia techniques

Lump - A mass of tissue that may or may not be cancerous

Lumpectomy - Surgery to remove a cancerous tumor from the breast. Lumpectomy is also called "partial mastectomy," "breast conserving"

Lymph Nodes - Small, round, or bean-shaped masses of tissue. They are part of the lymphatic system that helps your body fight infection and disease. As lymphatic fluid travels through the body, immune cells (called lymphocytes) in the lymph nodes trap bacteria, viruses, and other potentially harmful substances and destroy them to help prevent their spread. They also keep fluid balance in check.

Male breast Cancer - Male breast cancer occurs when malignant cells form in the tissues of the breast. Any man can develop breast cancer, but it is most common among men who are 60 – 70 years of age. About one percent of all breast cancers occur in men. About 2,000 men are diagnosed with breast cancer annually, with about 450 deaths due to male breast cancer occurring each year.

Many men may be surprised to learn that they can get breast cancer. Men have breast tissue that develops in the same way as breast tissue in women, and is susceptible to cancer cells in the same way. In girls, hormonal changes at puberty cause female breasts to grow. In boys, hormones made by the testicles prevent the breasts from growing.

Breast cancer in men is uncommon because male breasts have ducts that are less developed and are not exposed to growth-promoting female hormones.

Just like in women, breast cancer in men can begin in the ducts and spread into surrounding cells. More rarely, men can develop inflammatory breast cancer or Paget's disease of the nipple, which happens when a tumor that began in a duct beneath the nipple moves to the surface. Male breasts have few if any lobules, and so lobular carcinoma rarely, if ever, occurs in men.

Men should also be aware of gynecomastia, the most common male breast disorder. Gynecomastia is not a form of cancer, but does cause a growth under the nipple or areola that can be felt, and sometimes seen. Gynecomastia is common in teenage boys due to hormonal changes during adolescence, and in older men, due to late-life hormonal shifts. Certain medications can cause gynecomastia, as can some conditions, such as Klinefelter syndrome. Rarely, gynecomastia is due to a tumor. Any such lumps should be examined by your doctor.

Mammogram - The x-ray of the mammary gland, called a mammogram, aims to screen for breast cancer or to specify the diagnosis of an anomaly detected by a clinical breast exam.

Mastectomy - Surgical removal of part or the entire breast

Metastatic breast cancer (MET-uh-STAT-ik) - Metastatic breast cancer occurs when cancer cells spread to another part of the body. Breast cancer can be metastatic at the time of diagnosis, or following treatment. Cancer cells can travel through the bloodstream and spread to other organs and parts of the body.

The most common sites of metastases are the breast or area where the breast used to be, the chest wall, the lymph nodes, the bones, the lungs or around the lungs, the liver or the brain. If you have been treated for breast cancer and now have cancer cells in any of these areas, it is most likely breast cancer that has spread.

Metastatic breast cancer is different to recurrent breast cancer. Recurrent breast cancer is cancer that returns to the same part of the same breast after treatment, rather than to other parts of the body. When cancer develops in the second breast, it is almost always a new cancer, not a recurrence

Multiple Sclerosis - an inflammatory disease in which the insulating covers of nerve cells in the brain and spinal cord are damaged. This damage disrupts the ability of parts of the nervous system to communicate, resulting in a wide range of signs and symptoms, including physical, mental, and sometimes psychiatric problems

Needle Guided Biopsy - removal of fluid, cells, or tissue with a neddle for examination under a microscope. There are two types: fine-needle aspiration (FNA) and core biopsy.

Oncologist - A doctor who is specially trained in the diagnosis and treatment of cancer. *Medical oncologist* specialize in the use of chemotherapy and other agents-such as antibodies, hormones, etc-too treat cancer. *Radiation oncologists* specialize in the use of x-rays (radiation) to kill tumors. *Surgical oncologist* specialize in performing operations to treat cancer.

Oncology - Oncology (from the Ancient Greek ὄγκος *onkos*, "bulk, mass, or tumor", and the suffix -λογία -*logia*, "study of") is a branch of medicine that deals with cancer. A medical professional who practices oncology is an *oncologist*. Oncology is concerned with:

- The diagnosis of any cancer in a person (pathology)
- Therapy (e.g. surgery, chemotherapy, radiotherapy and other modalities)
- Follow-up of cancer patients after successful treatment
- Palliative care of patients with terminal malignancies
- Ethical questions surrounding cancer care
- Screening efforts:
    - of populations, or
    - of the relatives of patients (in types of cancer that are thought to have a hereditary basis, such as breast cancer)

Grade - of a tumor refers to how abnormal the cancer cells look under a microscope and how quickly the tumor is likely to grow and spread. The pathologist determines the grade of the tumor using tissue removed for biopsy. The following grading system may be used for adult brain tumors: **Grade I** The tumor grows slowly, has cells that look similar to normal cells, and rarely spreads into nearby tissues. It may be possible to remove the entire tumor by surgery. **Grade II** The tumor grows slowly, but may spread into nearby tissue and may become a higher-grade tumor. **Grade III** The tumor grows quickly, is likely to spread into nearby tissue, and the tumor cells look very different from normal cells. **Grade IV** The tumor grows very aggressively (fast Growing), has cells that look very different from normal cells, and is difficult to treat successfully. The chance of recovery (prognosis) and choice of treatment depend on the type, grade, and location of the tumor and whether cancer cells remain after surgery and/or have spread to other parts of the brain

Ovidrel – a brand name medication included in a group of medications called Gonadotropins. Gonadotropins (or glycoprotein hormones) are protein hormones secreted by gonadotrope cells of the anterior pituitary of vertebrates. This is a family of proteins, which are central to the complex endocrine system that regulates normal growth, sexual development, and reproductive function.

Radiation - A form of cancer treatment that uses high levels of radiation to kill cancer cells or keep them from growing and dividing -- while minimizing damage to healthy cells.

Radiation Therapy (also called radiotherapy) - The use of high-energy radiation to kill cancer cells and shrink tumors.

Radiologist - A doctor who reads and interprets X-rays and other imaging techniques

Remission - Disappearance of the signs and symptoms of cancer. When this happens, the disease is said to be "in remission". Remission can be temporary or permanent, partial, or complete.

Stage - The extent of spread of a cancer. The stage is based on the size of the tumor and whether the cancer has spread. These are the stages of breast cancer:
Stage 0 is carcinoma in situ (in place).
Stage I is an early stage of invasive breast cancer. The tumor is no more than 2 centimeters (three-quarters of an inch) across. Cancer cells have not spread beyond the breast.
Stage II is one of the following: The tumor in the breast is no more than 2 centimeters (three-quarters of an inch) across. The cancer has spread to the lymph nodes under the arm.
The tumor is between 2 and 5 centimeters (three-quarters of an inch to 2 inches). The cancer may have spread to the lymph nodes under the arm. The tumor is larger than 5 centimeters (2 inches). The cancer has not spread to the lymph nodes under the arm.
Stage III is locally advanced cancer. It is divided into Stage IIIA, IIIB, and IIIC.
Stage IV is distant metastatic cancer. The cancer has spread to other parts of the body.
.

Sentinel Lymph Node - the lymph node is first in the drainage system of an organ to entrap cancer cells. If the sentinel lymph node is found free of cancer, the likelihood of other nodes being full of cancer foes down tremendously, eliminating the need for their surgical removal and complications thereof.

Triple-Negative Breast Cancer (TNBC) - In triple-negative breast cancer (TNBC), the cancer cells do not contain receptors for estrogen, progesterone, or HER2. About 10 – 20 percent of all breast cancers are triple-negative. This type of breast cancer is usually invasive and usually begins in the breast ducts. Healthy breast cells contain receptors for the hormones estrogen and progesterone. They also contain receptors for a protein called HER2, which stimulates normal cell growth. About two out of three women with breast cancer have cells that contain receptors for estrogen and progesterone, and about 20 – 30 percent of breast cancers have too many HER2 receptors. Breast cancer that is estrogen receptor (ER) and progesterone receptor (PR) positive can be treated with hormonal therapies. Breast cancer with excess amounts of HER2 can be treated with anti-HER2 drugs such as trastuzumab.

In women with TNBC, the malignant cells do not contain receptors for estrogen, progesterone or HER2. Breast cancer that is ER, PR and HER2 negative cannot be treated with hormonal therapies or medications that work by blocking HER2, such as trastuzumab.

Fortunately, triple-negative breast cancer can be treated with other drugs, such as chemotherapy, radiation, and targeted therapies.

Tumor - An abnormal mass of tissue that's formed by an abnormal accumulation of cells. Normally, the cells in your body age, die, and are replaced by new cells. With cancer and other tumors, something disrupts this cycle. New cells are made when they're not needed, and old cells don't die. As this process goes on, the tumor continues to grow as more and more cells are added to the mass.

Ultra Sound - Diagnostic sonography (ultrasonography) is an ultrasound-based diagnostic imaging technique used for visualizing internal body structures including tendons, muscles, joints, vessels and internal organs for possible pathology or lesions

Ultrasound Guided Needle Biopsy - In fine needle aspiration biopsy (FNAB), the doctor (a pathologist, radiologist, or surgeon) uses a very thin needle attached to a syringe to withdraw (aspirate) a small amount of tissue from the suspicious area. This tissue is then looked at under a microscope. The needle used for FNAB is thinner than the ones used for blood tests. If the area to be biopsied can be felt, the doctor locates the lump or suspicious area and guides the needle there. If the lump can't be felt, the doctor might use ultrasound to watch the needle on a screen as it moves toward and into the mass. (This is called an ultrasound-guided biopsy.) Or, the doctor may use a method called *stereotactic needle biopsy* to guide the needle. For a stereotactic needle biopsy, computers map the exact location of the mass using mammograms taken from 2 angles. This helps the doctor guide the needle to the right spot.

This is a brief glossary of terms used in this book.

For more information, please visit

www.ericajhollomanfoundationinc.org

THANK YOU

For supporting Breast Cancer Chronicles by Erica J. Holloman, PhD

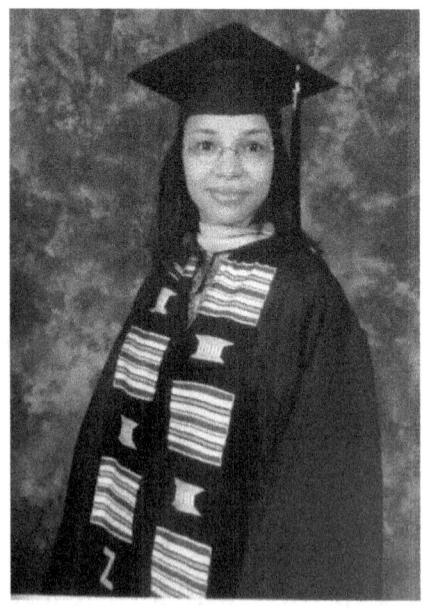

ALSO BY WAGNER WOLF

So You Wanna Be A Doctor??
The Untold Stories Of Medical, Dental, and Veterinary Residents

The Rich Must Die

Antoinette: Shattered Dreams

Blissful Encounters

...Pick up these great titles & more at WagnerWolf.com...

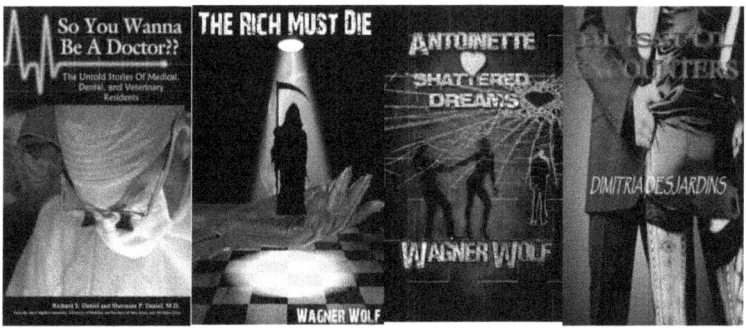

www.ingramcontent.com/pod-product-compliance
Lightning Source LLC
Chambersburg PA
CBHW071357170526
45165CB00001B/86